**Struggling for Health
in the City**

T0326545

Brigit Obrist

Struggling for Health in the City

An anthropological inquiry of health, vulnerability
and resilience in Dar es Salaam, Tanzania

PETER LANG

Bern • Berlin • Bruxelles • Frankfurt am Main • New York • Oxford • Wien

Bibliographic information published by Die Deutsche Bibliothek
Die Deutsche Bibliothek lists this publication in the Deutsche National-
bibliografie; detailed bibliographic data is available on the Internet at
‹http://dnb.ddb.de›.

British Library and Library of Congress Cataloguing-in-Publication Data:
A catalogue record for this book is available from The British Library,
Great Britain, and from The Library of Congress, USA

Published with the support of the Swiss National Science Foundation.

Cover picture: *Mama Afya* © by Brigit Obrist
Cover design: Thomas Jaberg, Peter Lang AG

ISBN 3-03910-673-2
US-ISBN 0-8204-7551-3

© Peter Lang AG, European Academic Publishers, Bern 2006
Hochfeldstrasse 32, Postfach 746, CH-3000 Bern 9, Switzerland
info@peterlang.com, www.peterlang.com, www.peterlang.net

Printed in Germany

Table of Contents

Acknowledgements   11

Abbreviations   13

Introduction   15

1   Household health practice and vulnerability   25
    1.1 Defining health   25
    1.2 Everyday conceptions of health in Europe   36
    1.3 Conceptualizing health practice   41
    1.4 The household as focal point of health practice   44
    1.5 Livelihood, vulnerability and health   54
    1.6 The health practice and vulnerability framework . .   61
    1.7 Study design and methods   66

2   Dynamics and diversity of city life   71
    2.1 Contemporary city life in historical context   71
    2.2 The informal sector, gender and social networks . . .   91
    2.3 Spotlight on an inner-city neighborhood   95
    2.4 Urban Swahili 104
    2.5 Discussion and conclusions 122

3   Everyday health conceptions 127
    3.1 Health definitions 129
    3.2 Health explanations 136
    3.3 Health activities 145
    3.4 Discussion and conclusions 169

4   Health practice within the household 175
    4.1 Negotiating responsibilities 177
    4.2 Receiving and giving support 211
    4.3 Discussion and conclusions 216

5   Health practice at the interface of household
    social groups, networks and institutions 221
    5.1 Organizing health activities 223
    5.2 Receiving and giving support 248
    5.3 Discussion and conclusions 256

6   Vulnerability to urban health risks 261
    6.1. Degrees of vulnerability 263
    6.2 Dynamics of vulnerability 269
    6.3 Interrelated dilemmas 299
    6.4 Discussion and conclusions 305

7   Health, vulnerability and resilience 311
    7.1 Health 311
    7.2 Vulnerability 317
    7.3 Resilience 324
    7.4 Conclusions 328

Bibliography 331

Index 355

Boxes

1   Newspaper clippings about major reforms
    in Dar es Salaam   87
2   Women's rationalizations why men
    avoid reproductive work 193

Figures

1   Health practice and vulnerability framework   63
2   Socially and culturally relevant response options 262
3   The interplay of urban health risks,
    response options and vulnerability 264

Maps

1   Tanzania and the location of Dar es Salaam   70
2   Dar es Salaam in the mid-1990s   96
3   Arial photograph of Ilala and Shaurimoyo   97
4   Street map of Ilala 228

Tables

1   Population growth in Dar es Salaam   77
2   Household structures 105

3 Religious affiliation of women and their husbands 111
4 Educational level of Ilala residents 113
5 Number of persons per room 114
6 Occupations of men and women 115
7 Dependence and headship 118
8 Descriptive definitions of health 129
9 Explanations of health 136
10 Health activities 145
11 Gendered responsibilities within households 178
12 Women's involvement in productive work 180
13 Dependence and women's involvement
     in productive work 185
14 Number of sick persons by social category 205
15 Health care decisions in relation to
     women's work patterns 207
16 Support in health practice within the household 211
17 Options for getting access to water 230
18 Receiving support beyond households 248
19 Providing support beyond households 252

Plates

1 Low-density, high-standard residential area 82
2 Medium-density, medium-standard residential area ... 82
3 High-density, low-standard residential area 83
4 Squatter settlement 83
5 Overview of Ilala Ilala 100
6 Swahili houses 100
7 A "contemporary house" 101
8 A neighborhood store 101
9 Traditional dress of Swahili women 109
10 Traditional dress of Swahili man 110

11 Preparing *chapati* 181
12 Plaiting hair 182
13 Baking a birthday cake 191
14 Cooking a family meal 192
15 Washing dishes 197
16 Doing the laundry 198
17 Ironing clothes 198
18 Bathing the baby 200
19 Grooming small children 201
20 Taking a bath in the *karo* 201
21 Getting ready for nursery school 202
22 Dressed up for nursery school 202
23 Grandmother as child minder 203
24 Fetching water 230
25 A street vendor selling water 231
26 Separating garbage 237
27 A garbage collector 238
28 City Council cesspit truck 239

Appendices

1 Geographic and ethnic origin of married women
(N = 93) and their husbands 349
2 Social characteristics of wives and husbands
in sub-sample (N = 20) 352

Acknowledgements

This book is based on longer and shorter spells of field research in Dar es Salaam over the past decade. I thank all the participants in these various studies and feel especially indebted to the residents of Ilala Ilala for their generous hospitality. My projects would not have been possible without my mentors and partners at the Dar es Salaam Urban Health Project, especially Dr. D. Mtasiwa, Dr. P. Kilima, Dr. L. Cloutier and P. Pichette, and the Department of Sociology and Anthropology at the University of Dar es Salaam, particularly Prof. R. Maghimbi and Dr. P. Masanja. My Tanzanian colleagues and field researchers, particularly S. Mlangwa, Dr. H. Minja, Dr. M. Mbilima and Dr. C. Mayombana with his team, kept my compassion alive and provided intellectual and practical support over all these years.

In Switzerland, my special thanks go to Prof. M. Tanner (Swiss Tropical Institute) and Prof. em. M. Schuster (Institute of Social Anthropology at the University of Basel) for their inspiring encouragement to carry these studies forward and submit an earlier version as habilitation thesis to the Philosophic-Historical Faculty of the University of Basel. I also thank the other referees, Prof. T. Harpham (South Bank University) and Prof. R. Wecker (University of Basel) for their valuable inputs. The Swiss National Science Foundation funded the main body of research on urban health practice as well as some of the smaller studies. My understanding of the complexities of urban health has been further enriched by two programs I was able to coordinate: the Ph.D. Program "Urban Health in Developing Countries" funded by the Swiss National Science Foundation and the University of Basel (1999–2002), and the Program "Vulnerability to Urban Health Risk" within the Individual Project 4 "Health and Well-being" of the NCCR "North-South: Research Partnerships for Mitigating

Syndromes of Global Change" funded by the Swiss National Science Foundation and the Swiss Development Corporation (2001–2005).

I also highly appreciate the support of Prof. L. Manderson during my stay at the Australian Center for International and Tropical Health and Nutrition, University of Queensland Medical School, in Brisbane, Australia. My colleagues at the Institute of Social Anthropology at the University of Basel and at the Swiss Tropical Institute have also aided me in intellectual and practical ways. I am very grateful to Dr. N. Stephenson and Ms. N. Stephenson for the English corrections as well as Ms. Z. Majapa and Dr. H.-J. Dilger for the Swahili corrections. Finally I owe a great debt to my husband and colleague, Dr. P. van Eeuwijk, for his critical mind, practical support and patience throughout this undertaking.

Abbreviations

AMMP	Adult Mortality and Morbidity Project
CCM	Chama Cha Mapinduzi (Revolutionariy Party)
DAWASA	Dar es Salaam Water and Sewerage Authority
DHS	Demographic and Health Survey
DSM	Dar es Salaam
DUHP	Dar es Salaam Urban Health Project
IEC	Information, Education, Communication
INHC	National Housing Corporation
NUWA	National Urban Water Authority
TANU	Tanganyika African National Union
Tsh	Tanzania Shilling (in 1995: 1 US\$ = 500 Tsh, in 2005: 1 US\$ = 1000 Tsh)
TzPPA	Tanzania Participatory Poverty Assessment
UNDP	United Nations Development Program
WHO	World Health Organization

If not otherwise indicated, the ethnographic present refers to the mid-1990s.

Introduction

Staying healthy in Dar es Salaam is a daily struggle. Like many other cities in developing countries,[1] the *de facto* capital of Tanzania has rapidly grown over the past decades. This urban growth, however, was not accompanied by economic growth. On the contrary, the country went through a deep economic crisis in the 1980s, followed by a Structural Adjustment Program in the 1990s, initiating rapid economic and political reforms. Rural poverty has driven people to the city and keeps them there, although most of them can barely earn a livelihood. What does health mean for people living under such conditions, and what do they do to maintain it? These questions form the core of this study.

Urban health research

Urban health problems are, of course, neither new nor restricted to Dar es Salaam. In the 1980s, a growing number of researchers working in cities of developing countries became concerned about the combined impact of the worldwide economic recession and rapid urban growth on people's health (Harpham et al. 1988, Salem and Jeannée 1989, Tabibzadeh et al. 1989). They have shown that these developments have outstripped the capacity of city

---

1   Throughout this text we use the somewhat old-fashioned term "developing country" as a convenient abbreviation. We prefer it to other terms like the Third World or the South, although we are aware that each of these terms has its deficiencies.

administrations and led to a veritable crisis in many cities (WHO 1993). This crisis manifested itself in a fall of living standards, a deterioration in both the quality and quantity of services and a decline of the quality of the built and natural environment (UNCHS 1996: 89), also in African cities like Dar es Salaam (Stren and White 1989).

The proportion of urban dwellers has steadily increased from 30 percent in 1950 to 47 percent in 2000 and will probably reach 60 percent in 2030 (UN 2004). If this growth rate continues, there will be as many city dwellers in the world as people living in rural areas by 2007. More than two thirds of the world's urban population live in cities of developing countries.

Urbanization does not necessarily pose a threat to health, as the experience in many cities of rich countries shows. If, however, rapid urban growth combines with economic decline and mismanagement, city administrations are no longer able to protect city dwellers from natural and man-made hazards, including negative effects of globalization (Satterthwaite 1993, Harpham and Tanner 1995, Atkinson et al. 1996, GTZ 2001, Harpham and Molyneux 2001, McGranahan et al. 2001). What we observe today is, in fact, an "urbanization of poverty" (UN-Habitat 2003a).

Epidemiological approaches

The theory and methodology of classic social epidemiology have guided most research on urban health. Investigators relied on quantitative methods to describe the extent, nature and distribution of health problems in urban populations and to measure the health impact of various factors. Priority areas were the often great health differentials within and across cities, the synergy of risks, the double burden of infectious and non-communicable disease due to a more general epidemiological, health or risk transition[2], and health problems related to difficulties in the delivery or utilization of health care and social services. Over the past decade, knowledge on urban health problems, especially in the four priority areas just mentioned, has greatly increased, and urban health has been put on the agenda of multilateral, bilateral and non-governmental organizations working in international health and development (Milbert et al. 1999). The Sustainable Cities Program of the United Nations Development Program and the Healthy Cities Program of the World Health Organization, for instance, have a strong focus on health (Harpham 1996, Pugh 1996, Werna et al. 1998), and both of them have become active in Dar es Salaam.

To highlight key issues in urban health research, we give a brief summary of a multi-country study carried out in Ghana, Indonesia and Brazil, more precisely in the cities of Accra, Jakarta and São Paulo (Songsore and McGranahan 1993, McGranahan and Songsore 1996, McGranahan et al. 1996). The aim of this study was to examine health differentials within and across these cities with a particular focus on the impact of environmental factors on diarrhea and acute respiratory infection in young children. Its findings document that conditions are worst in Accra, the smallest and poorest of the cities surveyed, and best in São Paulo, the largest and wealthiest. This means that the environment of a smaller city may be just as unhealthy as that of a mega-city, if inadequate household water supplies, bad sanitation, insect infestation, indoor air pollution and local accumulation of solid waste are common (McGranahan and Songsore 1996: 137).

---

2 The term "epidemiological transition" was originally defined by Omran (1971) to refer to the phenomenon of shifts in the relative importance of different diseases, basically a shift from infectious and parasitic diseases through receding pandemic and towards chronic, degenerative and manmade diseases. In developing countries and their cities, this health transition is delayed (Philipps 1993), especially among the poor (Heuveline et al. 2002). Recent reports promote the closely related concept of risk transition (WHO 2002).

Not surprisingly, the situation was found to be worst in poor neighborhoods of all three cities where centralized household services such as piped water, sewerage connections, electricity and door-to-door garbage collection hardly exist (McGranahan et al. 1996: 124). In these poor neighborhoods, local environmental problems are not only more severe, they also tend to reinforce each other to create a complex of interrelated environmental hazards. The synergy of risks increases, if members of different households have to share water sources, sanitary facilities and waste disposal services.

Even within poor neighborhoods, differences in environmental and health conditions have been established. In Accra, for instance, where the majority of the population is poor, if measured against international standards, and economic contrasts are muted, the study identified extremely diverse household conditions in terms of environment and ill-health (McGranahan and Songsore 1996: 148). In households with no or only one of the risk factors assessed by the study, the prevalence of diarrhea was also nil. As the number of risk factors increased, so did the prevalence of diarrhea. The same trend has been found for acute respiratory disease.

A crucial insight of the study is that more affluent households were able to shift both the intellectual and practical burden of environmental management to the government or a private service provider (McGranahan et al. 1996: 123–124). It can be inferred, in other words, that poor households have to carry a heavier burden in terms of environmental management than affluent households. They have to find their own solutions in terms of getting water, emptying septic tanks and disposing garbage, and this is not only a practical but also an intellectual challenge.

A new anthropological perspective

Many more studies could, of course, be cited, but this example is particularly suited to provide a background against which we can outline the theoretical approach of our study. Up to now, most urban health research has been informed by a view of health defined by experts and has concentrated on conceptual links between health, urban environment and poverty, conceptual links which were created by the theory and logic of the researcher. What health means to people who live in a particular locality, what links they create between health and other aspects of their reality, and what they do in their daily life to stay healthy are topics which have not yet been sufficiently examined in this literature. We do not simply refer to a distinction between "etic" and "emic" positions popular in the anthropology of the 1970s. At the centre of our analytical interest are individual persons as social actors who interpret experiences of everyday life and thereby construct and reconstruct meanings and values in interactions with others, and in particular social and cultural contexts (Hannerz 1992).

Our approach is guided by the theory and methodology of anthropology which, above all, seek to gain a better understanding of people and the meaningful world they create in different social, environmental and historical contexts. Drawing on the work of Michel Foucault (1963), Pierre Bourdieu (1977) and Anthony Giddens (1984) and their concepts of "agency" and "practice", we go beyond social constructivism and integrate a view of people as individual subjects and social actors with an analysis of cultural phenomena, social conditions and structural constraints. Such an approach, we argue, is particularly useful for the study of health and illness in heterogeneous and rapidly changing urban settings, where structural conditions force people to find their own ways of sustaining and restoring health. In an era of globalization, and especially in localities constrained by poverty, people have to use their reflective capacities as they confront new situations, contingencies, and uncertainties that interrupt the daily routine. We thus use a perspective that is resource-rather than deficit-oriented, not because of a calculated optimism, but in order to open a space for the consideration of people as actors, not victims, who shape their lives even under difficult circumstances.

In the field of urban health research, the need for such an approach has become increasingly recognized, particularly due to difficulties encountered in interventions. Tanner and Harpham (1995: 216), for instance, point out that technical solutions and standardized intervention packages alone cannot alleviate health problems. In fact, the best technological solutions help little, if they do not reach or are not accepted by the people and do not build on their resources. For this reason, Rapid Assessment Procedures[3] and Participatory Approaches[4] have become rather popular.

Following up on the multi-country study outlined above, researchers in Accra, for instance, used rapid assessment methodology to develop "proxy" indicators for routine monitoring of the environmental health situation in different neighborhoods (Songsore et al. 1998). In addition, the research team employed a combination of qualitative and quantitative methods to investigate the gender division of labor in and around the home and to assess gender and age differentials in environmental risks and resulting health effects (Songsore and McGranahan 1998). The

---

3   Rapid Assessment Procedures have been developed in order to make anthropological methods more useful for health research (see e.g. Manderson and Aaby 1992, Vlassoff and Tanner 1992, Obrist van Eeuwijk 1996). Among the first to provide guidelines for rapid appraisal in urban health research were Annett and Rifkin (1988).

4   Several books and papers discuss main issues and experiences in applying participatory approaches to health research (Vlassoff and Tanner 1992, Koning 1994, Koning and Martin 1996), urban studies (Mitlin and Thompson 1995) and urban health research (Guène et al. 1999, N'Diaye 1999, Odermatt et al. 1999).

findings of the qualitative component in the latter study indicate that male household heads are the key decision-makers in terms of allocation of resources to support environmental improvement, while women bear the burden of environmental management within the home. This creates tensions in the home which are further exacerbated by changes in the economic context resulting in a redefinition of gender relations. Moreover, the study found that the household is a socio-spatial construct of considerable importance in everyday environmental management, and so are networks of solidarity and other social and economic exchanges beyond the household.

The findings of this and of similar studies document that qualitative research brings to light the complex cultural, social and economic processes involved in environmental management essential for health on the household level. Based on such evidence, Harpham (1996: 5) suggests that future research should provide more insights into the social aspects of daily life and the experience of health and ill-health in the city, and Atkinson (1996) calls for an incorporation of "people-centered", "meaning-centered" and "power-centered approaches". What we need is a better understanding of the inner working of urban communities (Harpham and Molyneux 2001: 131).

The approach presented in our study claims middle ground between positivist and participatory epistemological stances (Obrist et al. 2003a). It is firmly grounded in ethnographic research in Dar es Salaam, an East African City in many ways similar to Accra in West Africa, and contributes to this innovative strand of urban health research. It develops an approach to study health practice with a focus on households, thus situating itself at the intersection of two major fields in the anthropology of complex societies: medical anthropology with its main concern for experiences, meanings and practices relating to health (Feierman and Janzen 1992, Good 1994, Nichter and Lock 2002) and urban anthropology with core interest in people's organization of daily life as individuals and members of households and social networks

(Sanjek 1990, Hannerz 1992, Gmelch and Zenner 1996). At the same time, our study draws on the somewhat disparate literatures of sociology, psychology, gender and development studies.

Overview of chapters

Chapter 1 argues that "health" on the household level is a fascinating new field for anthropological inquiry. Grounded in ethnographic field research as well as cultural and social theory, we combine approaches of medical anthropology and urban anthropology and link them with current debates in international health development. Health means different things to different people. We critically review various definitions and explain how we understand the concept in this study. Our focus is on health practice in everyday life, on social actors and moral subjects, who appropriate global meanings while facing the structural constraints of an African city. Emphasizing domestic health and vulnerability on the household level, we examine agency and resilience focusing on women from a gender perspective. We present our framework and outline, the study site and methodology.

The second chapter employs a historical perspective to identify the main forces shaping health risks and response options on the level of the city and the neighborhood. Particular attention is given to the urban health crisis of the 1980s and the fundamental political and economic reforms of the 1990s. We discuss the impact of the crisis and the reforms on the life of the city residents, abstract main features of urban social organization from previous research on survival strategies and fill gaps with new empirical data.

Chapter 3 narrows the focus on the household level and shifts attention from urban health risks to response options. It investigates health conceptions and their applications in everyday life from the perspectives of middle-aged women who belong to the lower middle class of Dar es Salaam.

The next two chapters examine the social dimensions of responses to urban health risks, especially internal household dynamics and connections with wider social networks. A detailed analysis of a gendered division of responsibilities in health practices enables us to identify social experiences as well as individual agency as women search for socially acceptable decisions and courses of action. We also critically assess meanings of support and the significance of reciprocity in a context of changing gender and generational relations.

Chapter 6 centers on the interplay of urban risks and response options from the point of view of individual women. Applying the health practice framework introduced in the first chapter and bringing together the different strands of analysis and argument developed in the subsequent chapters we assess how women put response options to more or less effective use. This allows us to group women according to degrees of vulnerability and to take a closer look at the dynamics of vulnerability in concrete case studies.

In the final discussion, we highlight the contribution of this study to different strands of research and outline implications for policies and interventions. Our qualitative study of vulnerability to urban health risks in Dar es Salaam provides a close-up view of patterns and differentials in women's health practice as they struggle to reach at least minimal standards of health while confronted with environmental hazards, commoditization, social fragmentation and, above all, the specific contingencies and uncertainties characterizing "informal cities" in rapid change. In this sense our findings have high inner validity for this particular locality. Generalizations based on ethnographic studies are, of course, difficult but our main findings tie in well with recent and on-going studies on vulnerability and resilience to poverty in Dar es Salaam and Tanzania.

1 Health practice and vulnerability on the household level

1.1 Defining health

In our Western societies, health not only constitutes a distinct conceptual domain, it has become a highly regarded value. Some even speak of health as a super-value (Crawford 1980: 380–382) or an idiom for talking about all facets of life (Becker 1995: 3). Just because of its high cultural significance, health remains exceedingly difficult to define.

In its Constitution of 1946, the WHO defined health as

> a state of complete physical, mental and social well-being, and not merely the absence of disease and infirmity (WHO 1967).

This notion of health emphasizes positive connotations, namely the presence of well-being, rather than the absence of disease or infirmity, and is broad in perspective, encompassing physical, mental and social aspects. Although this definition has been widely criticized, a broad concept of health has steadily gained ground. The sociologist Aaron Antonovsky (1979, 1987), for instance, developed a framework based on what he calls a "salutogenic" idea: it concentrates on what makes people stay healthy rather than what makes people fall ill. This perspective has also informed the rapidly expanding field of health promotion (Bunton and MacDonald 1992, Downie et al. 1996). Health, however defined, is now seen as a precious good, not just as something one has. This implies that one can do something to either lose or keep it.[1] Put

---

1 While public health specialists agree that health is more than the absence of disease, many would argue that an emphasis on positive dimensions of

differently, health means a quality one can put at risk, maintain or enhance.

Such a broad view of health, grounded in public health and epidemiology, has been widely disseminated and has become part of our general knowledge and popular culture. We see health as being influenced by a wide array of risk factors, and this shapes our ideas about personal hygiene, sanitation, smoking, exercise, diet and many other spheres of life. Increasingly comprehensive areas of individual existence and collective life have become subsumed under and validated as well as regulated by knowledge and practice grounded in medical and health sciences (Petersen and Lupton 1996). As Herzlich (1998: 176) has put it with reference to contemporary French society: Health is everything and everything is health. Not surprisingly, this phenomenon has been noted by researchers working in other European countries, for instance in Great Britain (Armstrong 1983) and Germany (Belz-Merk 1995), as well as in the United States (Crawford 1977, 1980, 1987) and Australia (Petersen and Lupton 1996).

Since the 1970s, ecological and environmental issues have gained increased recognition in the wider public, and this, in turn, has led to a new upsurge of interest in public health, not only in the wider public but also among experts. In the late 1980s, researchers postulated a New Public Health (Ashton and Seymour 1988) and claimed that the central concerns had broadened far beyond those of the "old public health" which focused

---

health is only justified in countries "where problems of high premature mortality are no longer a pressing social concern" (McDowell and Newell 1996: 12). Since this does not apply to cities of developing countries, experts study health through its negative dimensions. Using numerical indicators like morbidity and mortality rates, their main objective is to determine the frequency and distribution of disease and death (Robinson 1985, Rothman and Greenland 1998).

on "filth" and the control of odor, dirt and infectious diseases[2]. This widening of the perspective has also influenced research on urban health in developing countries. The WHO report entitled "The Urban Health Crisis" (WHO 1993), for instance, was written by John Ashton, one of the main proponents of the New Public Health. As the following quotation underlines, nearly all aspects of urban life are now examined in relation to health.

> Physical, economic, social, and cultural aspects of city life all have an important influence on health. They exert their effect through such processes as population movement, industrialization, and changes in the architectural and physical environment and in social organization. Health is also affected in particular cities by climate, terrain, population density, housing stock, the nature of economic activity, income distribution, transport systems, and opportunities for leisure and recreation. The impact on health is not the simple total of all these factors, but the effect of their synergistic action, the whole being greater than the sum of the parts (WHO 1993: 10).

In this view, health is a result of the complex interactions of people with each other and diverse aspects of the urban environment in which they live. A similar perspective has been formulated in studies on "population health" (Kindig and Stoddart 2003).

This broad view of health serves as a reference frame for our study. It directs our attention to what people in Dar es Salaam consider to be aspects of good health, to what they do to stay healthy, and to the links they see between health and everyday life in the city. Although these seem obvious questions to ask,

---

2   Public health originated in European cities of the mid-19th century and was constructed around the "sanitary idea" (Ashton 1991). In Victorian Britain of the 1840s, for instance, a public health movement formed around Edwin Chadwick as the guiding force (Wohl 1983). It was justified on the ground that the growth of the cities created enormous problems of sewerage and water supply and multiplied the risk of infectious and contagious diseases. Attention focused on "filth", a general term for the miserable housing conditions. Overcrowding in unsanitary conditions was seen as the root of the epidemics that afflicted the great towns and cities.

they have been neglected in previous research, not only in urban health research but also in public health and in anthropology.

Health behavior

If health behavior is investigated, it is measured against standards set by the biological and health sciences. In a frequently quoted definition health behavior is

> any activity undertaken by a person believing himself to be healthy, for the purpose of preventing disease or detecting it in an asymptomatic stage (Kasl and Cobb 1966: 246).

Although the conceptualization of health behavior has been expanded over the past decades (Alonzo 1993), it is still commonly seen as the corollary of biomedically defined risk behavior. The aim is to prevent certain diseases or to learn more about certain risk factors. This also applies to the more specific concept of "hygiene behavior" (Boot and Cairncross 1993, Curtis 1998). This concept refers to a wide range of actions that promote health, from eating a healthy diet to hygiene behavior associated with the prevention of water and sanitation related infectious diseases. Although various models and approaches are used in studies on health behavior, they all focus on individual perceptions (see Faltermaier 1994: 77). The analytical emphasis is on how individuals perceive their own susceptibility to illness, the severity of the conditions, the potential benefits of responding to recommendations, and barriers to health-enhancing action. The basic assumption is that individuals decide how to respond to recommendations made by a health care service by reflecting on the costs and benefits of such action in the context of how threatened they feel.

The anthropologist Mary Douglas (1992: 11) pointed out that psychologists studying risk perceptions place the focus on individual cognition and say practically nothing about intersubjectivity, consensus making, or social influences on decisions. These, however, are the most important aspects from an anthropological perspective. No one takes a decision that involves costs without consulting neighbors, family, or work friends. These people, on one hand, form the support group that will help if things go wrong. On the other hand, they tend to give conflicting advice. One of the interesting questions in risk studies would thus be to know how consensus is reached. In another passage, Douglas critically remarked that, in psychology,

> [p]ublic risk perception is treated as if it were the aggregated response of millions of private individuals. Among other well-known fallacies of aggregated choice, it fails to take account of persons' interactions with one another, their advice to one another, their persuasions and intersubjective mobilization of belief (Douglas 1992: 40).

Her argument is not against the reality of risks but emphasizes that people construct their interpretations and responses to these risks in social interaction. The conception of risk, Douglas contends, is a social and cultural construction, a fact not acknowledged by risk analysts committed to methodological individualism and mathematical probability theory.[3]

"Health" in anthropological perspective

Our approach builds on this critique. It does not investigate individual health perceptions and evaluate health behavior or hygiene behavior. Drawing on anthropological theory, its premise is that people's notions and practices relating to "health" and "risk" are produced and reproduced in social interaction. Our

3   An earlier book by Douglas and Wildavsky (1982) on the social and cultural construction of risk already received wide critical attention (see Johnson and Covello 1987). The ideas of Douglas have been further developed by Lupton (1999) who examines links between the conceptualization of risk and reflexive modernization.

analytical interest centers on how people explain good health and health practice, on which available meanings they draw, and how they interpret them as they relate them to their own experiences and life situations.

As mentioned above, this perspective has not only been neglected in public health but also in anthropology. Until now, most research in medical anthropology has been guided by the premise that "people become only aware of health in its absence" (Das 1990: 27) and that health can best be studied through its negative dimension – that is illness. This emphasis on illness is mirrored in the anthropological literature of the past decades, as several reviews demonstrate (Fabrega 1972, Young 1982, Good 1994).

Early definitions of the field of medical anthropology (Caudill 1953, Polgar 1962, Scotch 1963) were still broad in perspective. Polgar, for instance, included sections on "the healthy body" and "popular health behavior" reporting empirical evidence from an emic perspective. In these formative years, there were discussions about defining the field as "ethnomedicine" or "anthropology of health", but the term "medical anthropology" prevailed (McElroy 1996).

The narrow "medical" perspective is also dominant in studies carried out in cities of Latin America, Africa and Asia (e.g. Press 1971, Chavunduka 1978, Kleinman 1980), along the Swahili Coast in East Africa (Swartz 1991, Larsen 1998) and in Dar es Salaam (M.-L. Swantz 1986, L. Swantz 1990).

A partial exception are the proponents of "critical medical anthropology" (Singer and Baer 1995). They often use the term health in a positive sense but mainly as a goal that is difficult to reach under present conditions. Their aim is to identify and analyze the political and economic forces, including the exercise of power, that shape health, disease, illness experience and health care. Studies of this and of similar theoretical orientations pay particular attention to historical and political processes which are, in a large part, responsible for prevailing health conditions, for instance in a shantytown of northeastern Brazil (Scheper-Hughes 1992) or in various parts of Africa (Feierman and Janzen 1992).

There is also a body of literature which has tried to overcome the limitations of psychological and sociological modeling of health behavior and hygiene behavior by rich ethnographic research into the utilization of preventive services (Coreil and Mull 1990, Nichter and Nichter 1996). Even though our own perspective shares this concern, it follows another orientation. Our analytical focus is on people's everyday conceptions of health and health sustaining practices in their own right, not only in response to preventive services.

Massé (1995) recently argued for an "anthropology of health" *(Anthropologie de la Santé)*. He defined it as the analysis of the ways in which people, in diverse cultures and diverse social groups within cultures, recognize and define their health problems, treat people who are ill, and protect health (Massé 1995: 15). He calls for an anthropological account that puts more emphasis on health that constitutes the initial state, the positive reference *(référent)* that one wishes to maintain or restore. The domain of health, in his view (Massé 1995: 20), also comprises illness representations but, in addition, encompasses meanings and practices related to health protection. Most of the ethnographic material he discusses, however, focuses on illness.

Indeed, few anthropologists have produced empirical data on health as a discrete and positive notion. From the scattered ethnographic references available, we can infer that few if any societies had a generic term for a concept corresponding to our contemporary notion of health. The literature often mentions broader concepts like "balance" and "order" which go far beyond, but encompass, our positive notion of health. Especially the extensive anthropological literature about humoral traditions in Asia (Leslie 1976, Leslie and Young 1992), Latin America (Foster 1994) and Africa (Janzen 1997) documents culturally specific guidelines for achieving a balance or order.[4] These rules, however, are usu-

---

4   Some of these humoral traditions go back to the Greek scholars Hippokrates and Galen (Foster 1994: 12–13). Arab philosophers and physicians sys-

ally described in their "negative" form as rules for restoring health in times of illness, not as rules for sustaining health. This reflects, at least in part, the researchers' interest in medical systems, health care and therapy rather than health maintenance, but it may also indicate that people in many societies did not conceptually elaborate what they considered as normal.

In his study of the Swahili in Mombasa, Kenya, for instance, Swartz (1991, 1997) found most concepts concerning health, body functioning and illness to be similar or identical to those of Medieval Islamic theory and other Muslim communities. In this framework, the four humors "hot" *(bari)* and "cold" *(baridi)*, "moist" *(rughtba)* and "dry" *(yabisi)* are present in the body of every person, and they are associated with the four elements which make up the universe (fire, air, water and earth). The humors are differently affected by different foods – which are symbolically classified as "hot" and "cold". Each person has his or her unique balance *(mizani)* of humors which is linked with his character *(tabia)*, and as long as this balance is maintained, the person is healthy (Swartz 1997: 100–101). In the account of Swartz, this humoral theory was referred to in times of illness, and it was mainly formulated by healers and particularly knowledgeable individuals and known only in reduced form to the general public.

A different notion of "balance" as an organizing idea for health, sickness and healing has been reported from areas of Africa which were not transformed by the Islamic humoral tradition (Janzen 1997: 276). In many societies, „balance" referred to a

---

tematized and elaborated Greek humoral learning in Alexandria. With the Moslem expansion, the Greco-Arabic humoral tradition came to Western Europe and also spread eastwards. In Europe, this tradition became integrated into scholastic philosophy (Schipperges 1987), and from Europe, Christian colonists carried this legacy to South America. In Europe, humoral theory continued to dominate until the Enlightenment established health and the body as objects of rational inquiry (Labisch 1992).

broader notion of harmonious relations with other human beings, nature and the super-natural world. For the Zulu of South Africa, for instance, health of the body was only one aspect of good fortune in a more religious or moral sense.

> A Zulu conceives good health not only as consisting of a healthy body, but as a healthy situation of everything that concerns him. Good health means the harmonious working and coordination of his universe (Ngubane 1977: 27–28). […] In other words, I am using the English word "balance" to mean "moral order" in the symmetrical sense in relation to the position of people vis-à-vis other people, the environment, the ancestors and other mystical forces that produce pollution. "Balance" in this sense should be understood to mean "symmetry" or "order" rather than, as usual, the central pivot in a counter-poise situation (Ngubane 1977: 27).

Ngubane, an anthropologist of Zulu origin, refers to abstract European notions of "balance" and "moral order" in her interpretation of local concepts and practice. The Zulu did not have a word for balance, but the notion was implied in several words, particularly in *ukuzilungisa* meaning "to restore order where there has been disorder" (Ngubane 1977: 27).

Drawing on research among the Yole of Uganda over a period of thirty years, Whyte (1997: 13–14) makes an interesting point: People express a vision of a good life when they address ancestors and spirits. For the Yole, to be blessed is to have prosperity, marriage, children and peace, that is tranquility, well-being and freedom from worry. They also desire health *(obulamu)*, using a word which means life and, in a broader sense, comprises all the other blessings.

Based on these and other references we suggest that most societies with indigenous world views, that is world views not derived from European or other written traditions, did not have a notion corresponding with our concept of health which is primarily defined with reference to the human body. To be healthy was not seen as an objective in itself. The pursuit of health was embedded in a general pursuit of a good life and prosperity in economic, social, religious and moral terms.

Does this mean that anthropologists cannot study positive notions of health from the people's points of view? Such a stance seems hardly plausible in view of the transformations caused by colonial rule, international health development and globalization. Until now, anthropologists have commonly investigated whether and in what ways biomedical knowledge has become one of the frameworks in which people, even in remote corners of the world, have come to interpret misfortune, affliction and illness. They have compiled a large body of literature documenting how people move easily between different frameworks in their "quest for therapy" (Janzen 1978), using them sequentially or in parallel fashion for particular purposes. Directing their interest to the "health seeking process" (Chrisman 1977), they saw "the very work of construction, involving the use of disparate elements, assembled from various traditions as the afflicted family sees fit" (Whyte 1989: 293).

What has been neglected in anthropological research is that, as part of the same historical and political processes, the public health discourse has been taken up and spread through various institutional arrangements and has thus become one of the frameworks for interpreting fortune, prosperity and health.[5] In his social history of hygiene in Zimbabwe, for instance, Burke (1996: 17–62) has shown that it was mainly the missions, and, later, the state and civic groups which began to educate children and women in cleanliness and discipline, simple hygiene and sanitation. By the mid-1930s, a pedagogy of cleanliness and manners had become a standard part of school education in Zimbabwe, and various programs focused on generating new practices of domesticity and female behaviour. In the 1940s, hygiene training and domesticity were gradually taken over by women's organizations which, in the 1950s and 1960s, built up a broad movement with clubs and popular radio programs. This movement, according to Burke (1996: 62), solidified European-inspired ide-

---

5   There are, of course, notable exceptions, also in anthropology, for instance Manderson's (1996) study of health and illness in colonial Malaya.

als about hygiene and domesticity into a shared and collectively reproduced form of "common sense".

This example suggests that various institutions have contributed to gradually establishing health as a distinct set of knowledge and practice in Zimbabwe. We would expect that messages disseminated through education have created conceptual links between health and cleanliness, basic hygiene, sanitation and other aspects of daily life. Even if such conceptual links had existed before European intervention, they are bound to have been filled with new meaning derived from knowledge and practice grounded in the biological and health sciences.

As we pointed out earlier, an integral part of the public health discourse is the idea that people can influence their health. They can do something to maintain it, to put it at risk or to improve it. In Europe, the citizen's duty of maintaining health on the domestic level was largely represented as the responsibility of women (Petersen and Lupton 1996: 94). As Burke's study exemplifies, this social and cultural construction of women as main caretakers of health on the household level has been carried to Zimbabwe. It is, of course, true that most societies normatively assign reproductive labor to women, but Burke's findings indicate that this division of responsibility and labor has been reinforced and, at the same time, reinterpreted by the public health discourse.

Yet women in Zimbabwe were not only passive recipients of public health messages. As social actors, they have collectively reproduced European-inspired ideals about hygiene and domesticity in local discourse and practices. This issue has been increasingly emphasized in recent anthropological literature. A collection of studies about body technologies, for instance, exemplify that women's reactions to the process of "medicalization"[6] are

6   The concept of medicalization goes back to Foucault (1961, 1963) and Zola (1972) and their studies of medicine in Europe and the United States, respectively. It is commonly used to argue that biomedicine on behalf of the political elite has come to dominate previously independent traditions for

diverse and complex (Lock and Kaufert 1998b: 2). They found women's responses to range from selective resistance to indifference and selective compliance, but ambivalence coupled with pragmatism seemed to be the dominant mode.

These findings correspond with empirical data on local responses to globalization in many other social fields, documenting that dichotomies contrasting modernity with tradition, often implying colonial powers imposing modern technologies on traditional societies, are outdated metaphors (King 1990, Hannerz 1992, Appadurai 1996, Featherstone 2002). What we observe today are much more complex cultural processes of hybridization or creolization resulting in a great diversity of responses to the flow of ideas, goods and people around the globe.

1.2 Everyday conceptions of health in Europe

While anthropologists working in developing countries have shown little interest in people's conceptions of health, a few colleagues working in the United States (Crawford 1980, Saltonstall 1993, Arcury et al. 2001) have conducted studies on this topic, and a group of researchers working in Europe came up with a systematic approach. The French anthropologist and social psychologist Claudine Herzlich is a pioneer in this field. Herzlich (1969: 13–14) saw health and illness as a social representation,

----

understanding misfortune and well-being along with associated ways for alleviation or fulfillment. However, as the historian Merryl Vaughan (1991) has shown in her critical consideration of "Foucault in Africa", the concept of medicalization has to be used with caution in other cultural and social contexts. The discourse of British colonial medicine has, for instance, not been monolithic, unchanging or without its own internal contradictions (Vaughan 1991: 200).

that is as a complex construction through which the experience of an individual and the values and ideas of the society become integrated into a meaningful image. She developed her approach based on empirical, qualitative research in Paris and in Normandy. In long conversations she elicited people's accounts of health and illness and examined them with the method of content analysis. Here, we shall only report her findings concerning health.

Herzlich (1969: 79–89) abstracted three dimensions from her respondents' accounts. The first dimension, "Health in a Void" *(Santé vide),* implies the absence of disease. It refers to a state in which the body is silent, so to speak. The second dimension called "Reserve of Health" *(Fond de santé)* characterizes health as an asset rather than a state. Health is something one has, something that enables a person to perform a job. Physical robustness or strength and resistance to attacks, fatigue and illness are emphasized. The third dimension, "Equilibrium" *(Equilibre),* refers to "real health", to a notion of well-being which her respondents mentioned frequently but found difficult to explain. On one level they seemed to refer to a substratum of essential harmony and balance in bodily, psychological and spiritual life, on the other to what follows in a functional sense: self-confidence, happiness, having good relations, alertness, energy, and even freedom.

Three key findings of Herzlich's study have been repeatedly taken up in subsequent research:

– Different understandings of health and illness are not polar opposites of each other, but discrete conceptions. This means that the social representations of what makes a person healthy are distinct from those of what makes people ill.
– Lay people are able to express complex and sophisticated conceptions of health. Although distinct social representations can be abstracted from individual accounts, this does not mean that individuals use a single representation consistently. Most people rather recur to two or all of them, thus interweaving them into multifaceted conceptions.

– Health is seen as coming from within the individual, from his or her constitution, and individuals can take measures to protect and maintain health. Illness, on the other hand, is conceived as something external that is produced by the way of life and the society.

According to Herzlich's findings in France, the social representations of health constitute a distinct set of knowledge and practice. Subsequent researchers who followed her lead set out to investigate whether her findings were only valid for people with an urban middle-class background or also for people of other social strata. Qualitative studies in the United Kingdom focused on women of working-class background (Blaxter and Patterson 1982, Pill and Stott 1982, Pill and Stott 1985a, Pill and Stott 1985b, Pill and Stott 1987) or compared health concepts of women belonging to higher and lower social strata (Calnan 1987). They were complemented by quantitative studies in France (D'Houtard and Field 1984) and in the United Kingdom (Blaxter 1990).

Although these studies differ in terms of theoretical orientation and methods of data collection, some general trends can be outlined in comparison with Herzlich's conclusions. First, these studies confirm that people of different social strata in France and the United Kingdom are able to formulate discrete and complex concepts of health which draw on available meanings. The respondents described "positive" as well as "negative" – in the sense of grammatical form and content – dimensions of health in many different words and phrases, and they combined elements in many different ways.

Secondly, differentials in health concepts exist within and between social categories. In her survey, Blaxter (1990) found that definitions of health varied by stage in life cycle, gender and social differences. Younger men tended to explain health in terms of physical strength and fitness, older men focused more on being still able to do things, and younger women emphasized energy, vitality and being able to cope. People of middle age expressed ideas that were more complex and put greater emphasis on total mental and physical well-being. Better off and better-educated women formulated multi-dimensional concepts. In a similar vein, Williams (1990), based on a study in Scotland, argued that "old people" cannot be regarded as a unitary group who see the world in the same fashion. They interpreted the physical manifestations of growing old in a number of distinctly different ways. Still, his respondents shared a common account of health as strength. Within this account, health was seen as something that an individual person can "take care of", build up and maintain or, alternatively, spend or squander.

The findings of these studies indicate, in other words, that gender interacts with age and social differences based on education and occupation. Moreover, even within gender and age categories different, ambivalent and even contradictory conceptions of health may coexist. In more general terms, the studies provide additional evidence of an understanding of health as something which can, to varying degrees, be influenced by day-to-day conduct, either in a positive or negative way.

In the 1990s, a number of German psychologists began to investigate various aspects of health in everyday life (Flick 1991, Faltermaier 1994, Belz-Merk 1995, Strittmatter 1995, Faltermaier et al. 1998, Flick 1998). Most of their work builds implicitly or explicitly on the idea of health as a social representation which is experienced, defined and expressed differently by different social groups and in different cultural contexts. The research focus in these psychological studies is, however, on subjective notions of health which are examined against the background of various psychological theories.

Of particular interest to the present study is the distinction between three analytical constructs introduced by the psychologist Toni Faltermaier (1994, Faltermaier et al. 1998): health concepts *(Gesundheitskonzepte)*, health theories *(Gesundheitstheorien)* and health action *(Gesundheitshandeln)*. The first two constructs have already been referred to in the discussion of previous studies, but they have often been used interchangeably. Faltermaier suggests to use the term "health concepts" for understandings and descriptive definitions of health and "health theories" for explanations of what influences health. As a psychologist, his focus is 1) on *subjective* health concepts, that is on a person's understanding of health, particularly with regard to her own health, and 2) on *subjective* health theories, what a person sees as influencing her health (Faltermaier et al. 1998: 37).

What previous studies have not explicitly mentioned is "health action". Faltermaier (1994: 171–172) situates himself in the sociological tradition that goes back to Max Weber and his notion of "subjective meaning". By doing so he emphasizes the difference between his definition of health action and the concept of "health behavior" mentioned earlier. Health action refers to people's own explanations of potentially beneficial or harmful behavior and does not measure them against biomedical or public health standards. The aim is to examine people's accounts of complex and manifold daily activities of maintaining health in their own right. As a psychologist, Faltermaier puts his analytical focus on, at least partly, conscious, intentional and self-reflective behavior.

We argue that the systematic approach developed in these studies in Europe are also of use for research in Africa, but as anthropologists we are less interested in people's subjective health concepts and health theories, than in meanings created in social interaction. People talk to each other about experiences of health and illness; they exchange views and draw on available meanings. They consult with others, critically reflect on their advice and interact with them in the daily performance of health activities. Herzlich's view of health as a social representation comes close to our own analytical focus because it draws attention to how people's experiences shape and are shaped by broader forces of society, but her emphasis is on conceptions, while we are equally interested what people actually do in everyday life.

1.3 Conceptualizing health practice

For our analytical purpose, we suggest to move a step beyond a descriptive analysis and consider health conceptions as "health practice". As defined by Giddens (1979, 1984), the concept of practice[7] calls attention to what people do and to their capacity as human beings to reflect about what they do. In his view, practice implies two aspects of reflexivity. On one hand, people can describe, monitor and give rational accounts as subjects of their actions, on the other hand, much of what they do is embedded in tacit knowledge. Human agency, in other words, operates only partly on a discursive level.

> Human agents or actors [...] have, as an inherent aspect of what they do, the capacity to understand what they do while they do it. The reflexive capacities of the human actor are characteristically involved in a continuous manner with the flow of day-to-day conduct in the contexts of social activity. But reflexivity operates only partly on a discursive level. What agents know about what they do, and why they do it – their knowledge-ability as agents – is largely carried in practical consciousness. Practical consciousness consists of all the things which actors know tacitly about how to "go on" in the contexts of social life without being able to give them direct discursive expression (Giddens 1984: xxii–xxiii).

Giddens draws a distinction between "practical consciousness" and "discursive consciousness", yet emphasizes that this distinction is neither rigid nor impermeable. It only marks the differences between "what can be said and what is characteristically simply done" (Giddens 1984: 7).

This understanding of human agency and practice raises a number of important methodological issues. Anthropologists have

---

7   "Practice" has become a new key symbol of theoretical orientation, at least since the 1980s (Ortner 1984). It is neither a theory nor a method in itself, although Bourdieu (1977), one of the main proponents of this orientation, speaks of a "theory of practice".

long recognized that there is a "hidden logic" in people's ways of thinking and acting, and they developed various concepts to capture different aspects of this phenomenon, for instance "implicit meanings" (Douglas 1975), *"le sens pratique"* translated as "the logic of practice" Bourdieu (1990) or and "embodied knowledge" (Csordas 1990). Most anthropologists would agree that people's practices "encapsulate their values and their meaningful world" (Bibeau 1997: 249), and they use participant observation to gain insights into tacit knowledge embedded in the day-to-day flow of social life.

These theoretical considerations have interesting implications for investigations into health. By using the word health practice we suggest that people's health definitions, health explanations and health activities are rooted partly in enacted knowledge, partly in discursive knowledge. This means, in other words, that by asking people about health, we make them "switch" from practical consciousness to discursive consciousness, to reflect and talk about what they usually simply do. The same process, of course, occurs, if they themselves consult each other, if they ask another person about an explanation for something she has done, or if they face an unusual situation and discuss what should be done. Much of the routine of daily health practice, on the other hand, is embedded in practical consciousness, and so are shared meanings and understandings about health.

We can thus interpret health as a social experience which is enacted as well as verbalized. If we elicit people's accounts about meanings of health (health definitions and explanations) and what they do for health (health activities), we collect data on discursive knowledge; these should be complemented by observations of actual practice to gain an understanding of enacted knowledge.

Put differently, the concept of "practice" directs attention to the dialectical relationship of agency and structure. On one hand, human beings are agents or have agency in that they are capable of reflecting about available knowledge – whether it is enacted or discursive – and to act upon these reflections. On the other hand, individual actors are influenced by knowledge and other cultural phenomena, social conditions and structural constraints shaped by broader environmental, economic and political forces. While much theoretical and empirical research in anthropology emphasized the second aspect of the agency-structure relationship, interest in the first has greatly increased since the 1980s (Ortner 1984). Bourdieu (1977, 1990) uses the concept of habitus, Foucault (1961, 1963) the concept of discourse to capture the structuring of individual agency, as Giddens (1979) has called it.

If we see human beings as subjects of their actions who are influenced, but not determined by social experience and broader structural forces, we can record and examine how they reflect and thus give meaning to what they do. For such an analysis, Foucault (1984: 32–39) suggested to distinguish between three levels: 1) The code of values and rules which are prescribed to individuals and groups by institutions like the family, the school or the church; 2) the concrete behavior of an individual in relation to the prescribed values and rules; and 3) the way in which a person positions herself vis-à-vis the code of values and rules. From contemporary anthropological perspective, such an approach enables us to investigate how individual persons as agents reproduce and produce the social experience of health in daily practice.

Moreover, the study of the third aspect, Foucault argues, will show that the individual person is not just an actor, but a moral subject. Foucault developed this approach in his study of sexuality, a topic which clearly has a moral dimension. Although it is perhaps less obvious, we suggest that health does not only have a highly symbolic value, it also has a moral dimension. In spite of biological reductionism, many people, also in our own society, continue to see health as closely linked with ideas about a good conduct of life which are not only justified by the biological sciences (Petersen and Lupton 1996). Even if a lay person believes or trusts in medical knowledge, she can usually not reenact in her mind how these facts were established. "Belief", "faith" and "trust" open a space for moral judgment about right and wrong, good and bad. This happens in a largely secular society, and it is even more pronounced in societies where religions provide one of the frameworks for interpreting health and illness.

For this reason we suggest that the three steps of analysis outlined by Foucault can also be used in research on health. Of particular interest is not only the second, but the third level because it tells us something about the "why". By investigating how people position themselves towards knowledge, values and rules prescribed to them by institutions like the family, the school, the church or mosque or the clinic, we learn something about their moral judgments of what is good or bad for health.

By moving practice and agency into the center of interest, we put our emphasis on individuals as social beings. Individual persons do not act in a social and cultural vacuum. They take other persons, available meanings, knowledge, values and rules, their personal interest and material circumstances into account as they respond to particular situations. The concept of practice thus emphasizes the dialectic relationship between agency and structure, between individual action and opportunities as well as constraints shaped by broader economic, political and social forces (Ortner 1984).

1.4 The household as focal point of health practice

If we consider everyday health practice as a domain that is not only personal or psychological but social and cultural, we have to study it in an arena in which people interact with one another as well as with the broader environment. In urban settings, the household provides such an arena.

Household health production

From a public health point of view, the household plays a central role in "health production" (Berman et al. 1994). It engages in a range of health activities such as infant feeding, child care, home hygiene and sanitation as well as home based diagnosis and treatment of illness. Households also make use of externally available technologies, information and skills, for instance by using preventive and curative health services or other forms of treatment, and by making financial investments in health such as home improvements or purchase of health related goods like a refrigerator, a new stove, or a water pump. From this perspective one can actually speak of Household Production of Health defined as

> a dynamic behavioral process through which households combine their (internal) knowledge, resources, and behavioral norms and patterns with the (external) technologies, services, information and skills to restore, maintain and promote the health of their members (Berman et al. 1994: 206).

The analytical emphasis in this framework is on the social process through which resources can be mobilized within and beyond the household to strengthen positive dimensions of health. In this sense, the household is seen as both a locale and as a normative social environment.

While it seems convincing to see the household as a node between the domestic and the public sphere, this framework has at least two limitations. First, it takes experts' interpretations of "health" and "health behavior" as a lead without clarifying whether people themselves see a link between these aspects of daily life and health. Secondly, its conceptualization of the household is not consistent. On one hand, households are described as actors that can maintain health or make choices about health maintenance. On the other hand, it suggests investigating in particular contexts what "household" actually means, what its role is in health maintenance and which internal and external dynamics influence it.

Defining the household

This ambivalence shows that the Household Production of Health framework has roots in economics – more precisely in New Household Economics – and in anthropology. As feminist anthropologists (Dwyer and Bruce 1988, Moser 1993: 20–25) have critically remarked, New Household Economics assumes households to operate as decision-making units in production and consumption and thus treats them as actors. Anthropologists, on the other hand, do not see the household as a corporate unit with the boundaries and the motivation of an individual (Wilk 1991: 34). Some anthropologists working in Africa even question the usefulness of the concept for social analysis because African "households" are internally divided and embedded in wider social and economic networks (Guyer 1981, Guyer and Peters 1987, Guyer 1997). Most anthropologists would agree that "household" – like "kinship", "marriage" or "lineage" – is a Western construct; whether it is meaningful in a given local context has to be investigated, not assumed.

In this sense, the household can be defined as

> a coresident group of persons who share most aspects of consumption, drawing on and allocating a common pool of resources (including labor) to ensure their material reproduction (Schmink 1984: 89).

A reduction to purely economic functions, however, is not satisfactory.

> In most cases, the primary basis for the cohesion of the household unit is in fact a set of social relations and mutual obligations that are defined by kinship or other reciprocal relationships (Borsotti 1981: 179–180, in Schmink 1984: 93).

Since the 1980s, feminist researchers have become increasingly interested in investigating the meanings of "household" in diverse localities because it is an important social, cultural and material context for much of women's lives (Brydon and Chant 1989: 1). In their view, the household is the focal point of a division of labor and responsibilities between women and men derived from the framework of social relations in the wider society (Brydon and Chant 1989: 8–10). They formulated their research interest mainly as a critique of the conceptualization of the household in the theory of New Household Economics with its implicit model of a nuclear household led by a male head and breadwinner (Dwyer and Bruce 1988, Moser 1993: 20–25). The evidence, arguments and debates coming out of this research orientation are complex, but four issues seem particularly interesting in view of our own study, namely the heterogeneity of household structures, the division of responsibilities and labor within households, the social dynamics of decision-making among household members, and the embeddedness of households in wider social and economic networks.

In the following paragraphs we illustrate each of these issues with findings from studies in various cities, especially from Mexico City (González de la Rocha 1994), Lusaka (Hansen 1997) and Cairo (Hoodfar 1997). Their findings help us to formulate questions regarding the social organization of health practice in Dar es Salaam.

Heterogeneity of household structures

Chant (1989) conducted a broad literature review of urban household structures in cities of developing countries. She found that heterogeneity rather than homogeneity in size, composition and residential arrangements is a typical feature and identified seven types of urban household structures. Nuclear households, consisting of a couple and their children, have become a common feature of urban social organization, and so have single-parent households headed by a woman. Especially the latter have received much attention in feminist scholarship.[8] Extended house-

8   Chant (1997) provides a comprehensive review of the literature. According to her, there is little dispute that the number of women-headed households is growing, but precise figures hardly exist. It is presently estimated

47

holds often form around nuclear or single-parent households, as relatives become attached; all members of an extended household share in daily consumption and financial arrangements. Nuclear-compound households are similar to extended households, but they form separate units in respect to daily consumption and finances. Single-sex households are made up of either only men or only women. In a mixed household, members do not have a family base; unrelated persons such as friends or work mates share a dwelling. Single-person households, for instance a young man or a widow, are also a common feature of urban life.

Chant's typology demonstrates the complexity and range of households in urban settings. Arrangements vary in terms of size, composition and the degree to which productive and reproductive tasks are shared. These findings have important implications for our study. They show that we first need to look for a locally meaningful definition of the household, investigate the range of structures which fall under this definition and then examine whether differences in household structure are relevant for daily health practice.

Internal divisions of responsibilities and labor

Homes can be divided in many different ways (Dwyer and Bruce 1988, Fapohunda 1988, Papanek and Schwede 1988), and it seems as if the economic crisis of the 1980s and 1990s has affected the internal organization of households in many cities (González de la Rocha 1994: 132–160, Hansen 1997: 102–106, Hoodfar 1997: 264–275). Although the specifics of the economy and its effects differ

---

that they make up one fifth or one third of the total household population (Chant 1997: 70). Urbanization is not consistently linked with rises in female household headship, although in certain regions, particularly in Central and South America, the process seems to be associated with growing numbers of women bringing up children alone (Chant 1997: 93).

from country to country, a general pattern has emerged. Gender models[9] often assign the role of main breadwinner and authority to men. A focus on lived gender relations, however, shows that even if men try to live up to this expectation, they often cannot fulfill it due to increasing economic constraints. Women often contribute substantially to the household economy, not always out of choice, but because they are forced to do so to make ends meet. This often aggravates the built-in tensions in the conjugal domain and makes men and women grapple with the question, how domestic life should be organized. If women become involved in income generating activities, they commonly have three options, namely 1) to carry the double burden of productive and reproductive work, 2) to delegate some of their domestic work to other members of the household, or 3) to change the household structure (Chant 1991: 9). The latter may result in an extension, if kin or non-kin members are invited to join a household to increase the labor force, or in a contraction, if children are fostered out to lower household expenses.

Our study will thus have to carefully examine how gender structures responsibility for, and performance of, health activities. Moreover, we need to pay particular attention to effects of the urban crisis discussed earlier (see Introduction). A crucial question is how health practice is organized within households in a situation where the infrastructure as well as the distribution and quality of services essential for health have deteriorated, husband's incomes have decreased and wives are forced to get involved in productive activities. The argument here is not that women's involvement in productive work is a new phenomenon. Women in many parts of the world have been engaged in agri-

9   "Gender model" refers to cultural representations, "gender relations" to lived experience. It is by now a well-recognized fact that gender models rarely accurately reflect male-female relations, men's and women's activities, and men's and women's contributions in any given society (Ortner and Whitehead 1981: 10).

culture, handicrafts and other productive work for centuries. The point is that, in deteriorating urban settings, growing numbers of women have started income generating activities because the husband's allowance did not cover household expenses.

Social dynamics of decision-making

The effects of changing economic conditions have also been at the center of debate in research on the dynamics of decision-making within households (Dwyer and Bruce 1988, Moser 1993). Some scholars have suggested that the wife's power of self-assertion relative to the husband increases when she is a wage earner (Oppong 1981), and they therefore advocate for the involvement of women into the labor market. Others hold the opposite view. They contend that the wife's power vis-à-vis her husband decreases when she earns money of her own because the husband then often keeps more of his earnings to himself rather than contributing to the household economy (Whitehead 1981). Changes in the urban economy thus tend to increase inequalities between husbands and wives, particularly among people with lower incomes (Hoodfar 1988: 142). A view which has become fairly widely accepted by feminist researchers is that fundamental changes of women's power of self-assertion cannot be based solely on increased income (Bruce and Dwyer 1988: 8, Moser 1993: 27). Other critical factors mentioned by these researchers include women's self-perception of their status and personal power as well as a political recognition of gender issues.

A gender analysis of the various degrees to which members of a household have a say in household matters draws attention to the concept of negotiation. The persons with whom women covertly or overtly negotiate are primarily husbands, but depending on the cultural setting, household structures and specific situations, they may be children and other members like parents, in-laws or siblings (Bruce and Dwyer 1988: 1). Researchers often refer to Sen (1990) who described the household as an arena of "cooperative conflict". On one hand, household members collaborate and face outside forces as a unit, harmonize their activities and thus act as a corporate group, and on the other hand, they may have conflicts of interest regarding the allocation of resources or the division of responsibility. It is important to mention, however, that researchers writing from a feminist perspective aim to discover hidden inequalities, while the women they study "do not consistently reveal a discomfort with their lot" (Bruce and Dwyer 1988: 8).

These findings imply that our study should focus on women's negotiations with other members of the household. Earlier in this text (see Chapter 1.1) we quoted Douglas (1992: 11, 40) pointing out that people rarely make decisions on their own, especially if costs are involved. They consult with others, receive advice, and try to reach a consensus. In addition to these overt negotiations, we can expect women to respond to the husband, children or relatives living in the same household simply by acting in certain ways. A focus on these interactions will allow us to investigate cooperation as well as conflict within domestic units.

Embeddedness in wider social networks[10]

Family ties go beyond household boundaries and reach across the city, into other towns and rural areas. In the city, loose-knit networks have replaced the corporate descent groups, the ideal

10   The term "social network" is often used as a metaphor to refer to a complex set of interrelationships in a social system. Some researchers have used it as an analytical concept in a more specific and defined way. The study of social networks in urban settings goes back to a study of Barnes (1954) in Norway and a study of Bott (1957) in Britain and has been used to understand the urban social organization in rapidly growing cities of Africa (Mitchell 1969) and Latin America (Lomnitz 1977) as well as among the urban poor in North America (Stack 1974). Informal exchange networks have also been shown to exist within formal systems (Lomnitz 1988). Over the years, network analysis has become more elaborate and quantitative (Schweizer and White 1998).

type of rural social organization (Gilbert and Gugler 1994: 163). A typical feature of networks is that they are invisible. They can only be abstracted from descriptive, narrative accounts or observations about specific social actions and interactions.

Contemporary researchers frequently refer to the classic study of social networks by Larissa Lomnitz (1977) in Mexico City. Her basic argument was that social solidarity based on reciprocal exchange is mobilized through social networks as a resource for survival (Lomnitz 1977: 204–205). This does not mean that the people she studied did not participate in market exchange whenever possible or economically convenient. Yet because of the structural insecurity that characterized their day-to-day existence, they had to complement market exchange with reciprocity, since, alone, neither of them could guarantee survival. The social networks Lomnitz (1977: 135–151) described include relatives as well as neighbors and friends, and provide reciprocal assistance in domestic life, for instance loans in the form of money, food or tools, and in family emergencies. Arrangements of sharing expenses and collaboration in domestic tasks such as cooking and doing the laundry seem to have been limited to what she calls "extended household networks" (Lomnitz 1977: 105,110).

Recent studies confirm that membership in a household and wider networks is a person's chief means of access to resources in an uncertain world, where neither the economy nor the state provide much security (Hoodfar 1997: 8, Harts-Broekhuis 1997, Moser 1998). Moreover, they have found that individual persons have different social relationships for different fields and different purposes (González de la Rocha 1994: 215). People do not see and relate to the same people for all activities. Couples tend to rely on a common network formed by the families on both sides, but individuals often have their own networks corresponding with the different niches in which women and men operate. In addition to women's and men's networks, these researchers distinguish between horizontal and vertical networks (Hoodfar 1997: 217–240). Reciprocity exchanges can occur between people and households with the same standard of living and social position or between individuals and households of higher and lower social economic levels.

Drawing on these findings, our study will have to investigate with whom women interact beyond the household. Since individual women may have different relationships for different fields and purposes, it will be important to examine their interactions with other persons for specific health activities. It will be interesting to see how women use social relations beyond the household as resources to overcome constraints imposed upon them by the urban crisis. We shall have to inquire into reciprocity, often mentioned as the organizing principle of social networks, whether they span horizontally or vertically.

Although feminist researchers criticize what they consider as a conventional view of the household, they agree that a focus on households is important for an examination of the social organization of economic life in urban settings. Despite its lack of unity, its greater or lesser impermanence and the extent to which inter-household ties are maintained with kin, friends or neighbors, they contend that the household is an important analytical concept. As Hoodfar (1997: 8) put it, most people go through life interacting with the wider society as members of a household rather than as autonomous individuals. Most importantly from the point of view of feminist anthropology, a focus on households "allows close scrutiny of the nature of gender relations and of the cultural and economic factors that help to bring about changes in them" (Hansen 1997: 95).

We also consider the household as an important focus of research and will examine the social organization of health practice on two levels: Within the household and beyond the household. For analytical purposes, we draw this line sharper than it is in reality. However, it seems important to determine the role of the household in day-to-day health practice because it is the key unit in many surveys and interventions. At the same time, we intend to draw attention to health activities that involve persons and groups outside the household.

1.5 Livelihood, vulnerability and health

Much of this research on urban households has been conducted to gain a better understanding of "survival strategies".[11] This concept, however, is controversial. "Survival" conjures up an image of life or death in the face of natural or man-made disasters like famine, earth quakes or cyclones. Even if life in urban environments is harsh, it is rarely that dramatic. Meanings of "survival" need to be examined in particular social and historical contexts since definitions of basic needs will vary over time, both within and between societies (Schmink 1984: 91). Moreover, some critics contend that there are no alternatives in the context of poverty and, without them, there are no decisions and hence no strategies (Selby et al. 1990: 66–71). Others argue to the contrary (Chant 1991, González de la Rocha 1994: 13): People living in material poverty have to seek and learn, to accommodate and adapt actions, and this involves convincing, helping, and forcing others to share work, give help and exchange favors. Such behavior implies options and strategies that may not be offered to the poor but are created by them.

In the field of development studies, many contemporary researchers prefer the concepts of "livelihood" and "vulnerability" to those of "poverty" and "survival strategies". This shift of perspective has been suggested by Robert Chambers (1989) who argued that the conventional definition of poverty does not capture the day-to-day reality of people living in developing countries. It is formulated in terms of low income or consumption in order to

---

11   Urban anthropology has a long tradition of studying the ways in which people living in poverty organize themselves to gain a living, particularly in Middle and South America (Lewis 1959, Lewis 1961, Lloyd 1979). The term "survival strategies" goes back to Duque and Pastrana (1973) and their study in Santiago de Chile and was popularized by the work of Lomnitz (1977) in Mexico City.

make it amenable to measurement. If people's lived experience is taken into account, additional dimensions have to be considered, such as livelihood and vulnerability.

Most people in developing countries, even in urban areas, cannot subsist on wage earning, either because they are unemployed or because their wage is too low. The concept of livelihood has been introduced to account for this fact. Not employment but diverse ways of gaining a living and security characterize the economic and social life of most people. Rather than undermining their efforts through policies and interventions focusing primarily on employment, people's ingenuity of making a livelihood under harsh conditions should be supported.

The concept of vulnerability emphasizes another aspect. In the definition of Chambers (1989: 1), it means "not lack or want but defenselessness, insecurity, and exposure to risks, shocks and stress". On the one hand, people living in disadvantaged environments are exposed to shocks, risks and stress (external side of vulnerability), on the other, they do not have the means to sustain a living without damaging loss (internal side of vulnerability). Loss can take many forms: Becoming physically weaker, economically deprived, socially dependent, humiliated or emotionally harmed. Vulnerability in this sense is the opposite of security. It refers to contingencies and stress and to the difficulty of coping with them (Chambers 1989: 1).

Chamber's definition has been widely quoted, and his approach continues to stimulate research, both in academic and applied fields, especially in studies on development, security and globalization (Bohle et al. 1994, 2001, Watts 2002, Krüger and Macamo 2003, TzPPA 2002/03). [12]

12 The concept of vulnerability has its own history in specific disciplines and fields. In medicine and epidemiology it often refers to biological and physiological processes, but due to the health (or risk) transition this understanding has broadened to include social and economic aspects, e.g. in research on adolescent health (Blum et al. 2002), HIV/Aids (Delor und Hubert 2000) and on other diseases of poverty like TB and malaria (Bates et al. 2004a, 2004b).

Urban vulnerability

Chamber's idea has also been further developed in studies on urban vulnerability in cities affected by macro-economic crisis. Caroline Moser (1998: 3) defines vulnerability as

> insecurity and sensitivity in the well-being of individuals, households and communities in the face of a changing environment and implicit in this, their responsiveness and resilience to risks that they face during such negative changes (Moser 1998: 3).

Although social and economic aspects of life are at the center of interest in this definition, the use of words like "well-being" and "risks", and in fact "vulnerability", imply that this discourse shares common concerns with that of the New Public Health and urban health research.

Further similarities between these discourses become evident, if we consider the main features of urban vulnerability identified by Moser (1998: 4), namely commoditization, environmental hazards and social fragmentation. In the urban economy, shelter, food, water and many other goods and services are commodities. People need cash to pay for them. One could say that the lower their level of income, the more difficulties they face in gaining access to basic necessities, and the higher their risk of destitution. The main environmental hazards Moser mentions are poor quality of housing and inadequate water supply, sanitation and solid waste disposal. With regard to social fragmentation Moser points out that greater social and economic heterogeneity may weaken community and intra-household mechanisms of trust and collaboration, especially under conditions of economic hardship. Urban health specialists, we have seen, consider even more aspects of urban life as having an impact on health, but their general orientation is very similar to that outlined by Moser in terms of urban vulnerability.

We suggest that research on what people do to stay healthy can learn from research on people's strategies to reduce vulnerability. The latter commonly focuses on "assets", on what poor

56

people have rather than what they do not have (Moser 1998: 1). It uses, in other words, a resource-oriented approach as the present study does but phrases its concerns in an economic idiom.

Based on her empirical research in Lusaka (Zambia), Guayaquil (Ecuador), Metro Manila (Philippines) and Budapest (Hungary), Moser developed an Asset Vulnerability Framework. Her central idea is to focus on assets, on what poor people have rather than what they do not have (Moser 1998: 1). This framework examines well-known tangible assets such as labor and human capital (health, skills, education), less familiar productive assets such as housing, and largely invisible intangible assets such as intra-household relations and social capital (reciprocity within communities and between households based on trust deriving from social ties). The crucial question in this research is how poor people manage these assets and how their management affects household vulnerability.

Although framed in a different language, such an approach addresses most of the issues discussed in the previous section. Regarding the asset labor, for instance, it examines the effects of the economic crisis on the division of labor between husband and wife and their consequences for intra-household organization. The aim then is to find out how people organize themselves to mobilize the asset labor, for instance by increasing the number of women working, by allocating the double burden of productive and reproductive work to women, and by increasing reliance on child labor.

In this framework, health is also regarded as an asset and classified under the category "human capital" (Moser 1998: 4). Other researchers guided by the same orientation (Chambers 1989: 4, Corbett 1989, Evans 1989, Pryer 1989) have argued that the poorer people are, the more it matters to be physically able to work and earn, the more they depend on physical work, and the higher are the personal costs of physical disability. At the same time, the poor face more obstacles in the improvement of health (asset accumulation). First, their bodies are more exposed to inadequate nutrition and to sickness from unsanitary, polluted and disease-ridden environments both at work and at home. Secondly, medical costs often exhaust the tangible assets of households. This has particularly severe consequences for all household members, if the breadwinner – whether male or female – falls ill.

Our study departs from these approaches in that it concentrates on one "asset", namely health. On the other hand, it will draw on these approaches by asking what assets or resources women mobilize in order to keep the family in good health and to reduce the family's vulnerability. Such an approach seems particularly useful to examine differences between households and to investigate, why some fare better than others.

This has been shown in another study on urban vulnerability carried out by the German geographer Fred Krüger (1997) in Gaborone (Botswana). Krüger was primarily interested in the complex relationships between livelihood and vulnerability, especially in housing, food security and health, and their differential impact on vulnerability. In a household survey, he identified economic and social risk factors which help to explain inter-household differences in exposure to vulnerability and then arranged them in a logical sequence (Krüger 1997: 237) to identify the position of each household.

Based on this analysis, Krüger (1997: 241–244) classified households into three groups. The least vulnerable households were comparatively well off, food provision and housing were secure, and they were embedded in social networks. Yet since each household was exposed to at least one of the risks listed above, there was a potential vulnerability to crisis. About 50 to 60 percent in his sample fell into this group. The middle range households had lower or less regular income, were exposed to two risk factors and occasionally had to fall back on agricultural resources or social support networks. There was an acute vulnerability to crisis because these households had no "cushion" to overcome critical life events or emergencies. This group made up about 25 to 35 percent of the households in his sample. The most vulnerable households had to combine a broad spectrum of resources to cover the daily needs, and they were exposed to three or more of the above-mentioned risk factors. Most of these households were tenants, and often a big number of dependents relied on one or two breadwinners. These households are already in an acute life security crisis, and their very existence is endangered. 5 to 15 percent of the households in his sample belonged to this group.

It is important to note that Krüger (1997: 241–244) classified women-headed households in all three groups, from least to middle and most vulnerable households. Some researchers have suggested that "the global economic downturn has pressed most heavily on women-headed households, which are everywhere in the world, the poorest of the poor" (Tinker 1990: 5). Others have warned against the stereotype view of women who run a single-parent household as "victims" of social and economic change (Chant 1991: 10, Chant 1997: 100). Krüger's findings provide additional evidence for this critical stance.

The model developed by Krüger will serve as a guideline for examining inter-household differences in health practice in Dar es Salaam. However, we modify his approach by focusing on "response options" rather than "risk factors". Based on our analysis of everyday health conceptions and task centered interactions, we will be able to identify locally available and socially acceptable response options women have. However, not all women (can) put these options to best use. After arranging the options along a continuum, we can then examine differences in women's use of these options. In a last step, we shall classify women into categories ranging from those that fare best to those that fare worst.

Vulnerability to poverty in Tanzania

The concept of response option has been introduced in a study on vulnerability and resilience to poverty carried out as part of the Tanzania Participatory Poverty Assessment (TzPPA 2002/03).

This policy-oriented study was conducted in thirty sites around Mainland Tanzania in 2002, including rural as well as urban communities, and both the conceptual framework and its main findings inform current policy making and interventions (United Republic of Tanzania 2003). According to the conceptual framework used in this study, people's vulnerability is a result of exposure to and intensity of impoverishing forces and effectiveness of their response options (TzPPA 2002/03: 13–29). It draws attention to the fact, that impoverishing forces can be sudden and unpredictable disasters like floods or droughts, but they can also be constant and sure, like environmental degradation, economic hardship or other stresses that reduce people's well-being. However, even when people face comparable impoverishing forces, they are not equally affected since they make differential use of response options. People operate, in other words, within the context of complex circumstances which sometimes facilitate and sometimes limit what they can do to avoid, overcome or simply live with consequences of impoverishing forces.

In this framework, impoverishing forces shape, but do not determine people's response options; just as important are assets people have at their disposal and factors limiting their use. As in the study of Moser outlined above, assets are mainly defined as various types of "capital", while the limiting factors have been grouped in two categories (TzPPA 2002/03: 23–25):

– Factors based on individual, household or community attributes: Access to assets, lifecycle-linked conditions, and hope.
– Factors reflecting the settings in which people live: Governance, economic conditions, environmental conditions, and socio-cultural conditions.

From a social science perspective, this is a very useful approach because it shifts attention to a better understanding of response options, the ways people (can) put them to (best) use. Like the practice approach, it emphasizes the complex interplay of individual agency and opportunities and constraints shaped by broader economic, political and social forces. Last but not least, it suggests a useful distinction of analytical levels which can help us to reduce the complexity of urban reality.

1.6 The health practice and vulnerability framework

Our framework contributes to these current debates by advancing and combining four principles.

1. We argue for a reorientation of medical anthropology as it is conceptualized in the Anglophone literature towards a health anthropology encompassing an anthropology of health and illness (see also Obrist et al. 2003a). Such a broad view has already been widely accepted in the Francophone world. Herzlich (1969) has emphasized that "health" and "illness" are discrete conceptions, not just polar opposites of each, and Massé (1995) has suggested to concentrate more on health because it constitutes the initial state, the positive reference that one wishes to maintain or restore (Massé 1995). These arguments are in line with various developments in epidemiology, public health and medicine advocating eco-bio-psycho-social models of health and a focus on health risks rather than disease. Such a perspective is particularly applicable to research on health in cities of developing countries, where people face a broad spectrum of health risks influenced by economic, environmental, political and social factors (Harpham and Molyneux 2001).

2. We understand health as a comprehensive concept which is closely linked to bodily, material, spiritual and social well-being, and define as its opposite not "disease" but "vulnerability to health risks". "Risk" and "vulnerability", like health, are multidimensional concepts and mean different things to different people. In this study, we draw on definitions which have re-

cently been developed in closely related research. "Risk" means the "probability of an adverse outcome, or a factor that raises this probability" (World Health Report 2002: xiii) and people's "vulnerability" is seen as result of exposure to and intensity of health risks in combination with the number and effectiveness of their response options (modified after TzPPA 2002/03: 18).

3. The guiding principle of our approach is the salutogenic idea of Antonovsky (1979, 1987). At the centre of our analytical interest is what makes people stay healthy rather than what makes people fall ill. This emphasis draws attention to individual persons as actors, not victims, who use their personal, social, cultural and economic resources to struggle for health even under constrained urban conditions.

4. Our approach, however, differs from positivist epistemological stances underlying most of the above mentioned public health and social science research including the work of Antonovsky. Rooted in anthropology and social and cultural theory, our framework encourages research that employs an interpretive perspective. It goes, however, beyond a position of social constructivism and focuses on the dialectic relationship between "agency" and "practice" (Bourdieu 1977, Giddens 1984). At the centre of analytical interest are individual women and men as subjects and social actors facing opportunities and constraints as they engage in interactions with other individuals and groups as well as with the specific cultural, economic and political contexts in which they live. In our view, this approach is particularly appropriate for research on health and illness in heterogeneous and rapidly changing urban settings, where broader political and structural forces have a direct impact on everyday life, but fail to create a space of material and spiritual security for sustaining and restoring health. Such constrained circumstances force people to use their practical, intellectual and emotional capacities to help themselves in their struggle for health.

The following chapters exemplify our conceptual framework which is firmly grounded in ethnographic field research. As visualized in Figure 1, our inquiry begins with an analysis of different phases of urban development which have shaped the dynamics and diversity of contemporary life, both on the level of the city and the neighborhood (Chapter 2). The aim is to identify broader forces which manifest themselves as urban health risks and/or factors limiting people's response options, especially with regard to environment, economy, government and society.

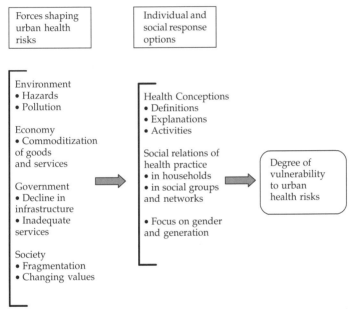

Figure 1
Health practice and vulnerability framework

The focus then narrows on individual and social response options in everyday health practice on the household level. We first concentrate on everyday health conceptions (Chapter 3). The question here is what kind of health knowledge people have and how they can put it to use in their daily life. Building on previous research in Europe (Faltermaier 1994, Faltermaier et al. 1998) we investigate local health conceptions, i.e. what people think and do about "good health". We go, however, a step further and reconsider these conceptions in terms of "agency" and "practice".

We then examine the social organization of health practice, first within households (Chapter 4) and then in social groups and networks (Chapter 5). The objective of these chapters is to get a better understanding of the social dynamics shaping response options through empirical investigation of actual health practice. For this purpose we introduce the concept of "task-centered interactions"[13]. This concept considers health activities as tasks, culturally assigned to certain categories of people by virtue of gender, household membership or another principle of social organization. Moreover, it implies that people interact with others when they carry out particular tasks. These interactions may take many forms and range from exchanging views and giving advice, over practical or financial assistance to negotiation, collaboration or delegation. The concept of task-centered interactions directs the empirical investigation of social dynamics and facilitates the mapping of relevant groups and networks on the local social organization.

This focus enables us to study gender from a women's perspective. Gender, as we understand it, is produced relationally within specific cultural, economic and political contexts (Lamphere et al. 1997: 4). As many researchers working in contemporary cities of developing countries have shown (see Chapter 1.4), the deterioration of the economy has forced women and men to reassess and renegotiate their relations towards one another and the wider society. We assume that this process of reassessment and renegotiation also affects the social organization of health practice.

---

13 In wording, not in content, this concept has been inspired by that of "theme centered interaction" (Themenzentrierte Interaktion) introduced by Cohn (1997) in the fields of group psychology and adult education.

A focus on task-centered interactions further enables us to examine health decision-making. Following Finch and Mason (1993: 60), our study argues that people's behavior cannot be explained by saying that somebody is following a social rule or obligation. Neither is a person's behavior explained straightforwardly by her position in the social world, for instance by the fact that she is a woman, a mother, and so on. By contrast, we argue that the course of action a person takes evolves from her interactions with other people. Decisions, we suggest, are a product of social interactions.

Finally, we consider the links between health and vulnerability, focusing on women from a gender perspective. Building on the analysis of the previous chapters, we identify a range of response options which may increase or decrease women's vulnerability. This enables us, on one hand, to analyze differentials in vulnerability across households and to divide women into categories ranging from least, to middle and most vulnerable. It also allows us to capture the dynamic nature of urban vulnerability: We select individual women from each category and document how their life situation changes over several months. These case studies provide a close-up view of how women put response options to use and thus either increase health and to reduce vulnerability in everyday life.

Our findings will show that this framework facilitates studies providing a scientifically informed basis for initiatives to support and improve health practice that are tailored to a particular locality. Moreover, it generates empirically grounded research questions and thus engages anthropology in current debates in research on urban health, vulnerability and resilience (see Obrist and Eeuwijk 2003, Obrist et al. 2003b).

1.7 Study design and methods

The study presented here forms part of ongoing research in Dar es Salaam.[14] Most of our studies have been carried out in collaboration with the Dar es Salaam Urban Health Project.[15] Data on health practice have been collected during an ethnographic study of eighteen months from 1995 to 1996 and a follow-up in 2002.

Our research site was an inner-city neighborhood. We selected this site because it is a planned residential area and considered as a lower middle-class neighborhood. Most previous studies have been conducted in squatter settlements. Moreover, it already served as a sentinel area for the large-scale Adult Mortality and Morbidity Project (AMMP)[16] of the Ministry of Health of the United Republic of Tanzania. By choosing this sentinel area, we

14 Various articles further elaborate aspects presented in this book (Obrist van Eeuwijk and Mdungi 1995; Obrist van Eeuwijk and Mlangwa; 1997; Obrist van Eeuwijk 1998; Obrist van Eeuwijk 1999a; Obrist van Eeuwijk 1999b; Obrist van Eeuwijk 2002a; Obrist van Eeuwijk 2002b; Obrist van Eeuwijk 2002c; Obrist van Eeuwijk and Tanner 2002; Obrist 2003; Obrist and Eeuwijk 2003; Obrist et al. 2003a; Obrist et al. 2003b; Obrist 2004; Obrist n. d.).

15 From 1990 to 2002, the Dar es Salaam Urban Health Project (DUHP), sponsored by the governments of Tanzania and Switzerland, improved the government health services and the health of the population in Dar es Salaam. The Swiss Tropical Institute in Basel, Switzerland, acted as the executing agency on behalf of both governments, in close collaboration with the City Council of Dar es Salaam. With the reorganization of the city government and administration, the DUHP has become integrated in the new City Council.

16 As the name implies this project collects data on adult morbidity and mortality and in order to do so, it set up a demographic surveillance system in 1992 covering a population of 307,912 in urban and rural areas. The urban project area is in Dar es Salaam, more precisely in Ilala, Keko and Mtoni. The two rural areas include Morogoro Rural District, approximately 180 km west of Dar es Salaam, and Hai District on the slopes of the Kilimanjaro in north-eastern Tanzania (see AMMP 1997: 18).

created cross benefits for the anthropological and the epidemiological research. The staff of the AMMP was interested in ethnographic data to learn more about the people "behind the figures" and to gain insights into people's daily life. Our study, on the other hand, could make use of the quantitative data collected through the demographic surveillance system, both in sampling and in the interpretation of our demographic data. We divided our study into several, partly overlapping components and employed a range of research techniques to investigate day-to-day health production in this neighborhood. The first component was a community study. It drew a profile of the selected neighborhood, its history, built environment, services, infrastructure and transport links and examined the government structure in which this neighborhood was embedded. Data collection was ongoing and included document reviews, interviews, group discussions, participant observation and casual conversation.

In the second component, the household study, we narrowed the focus on a purposive sample of 100 households. This sample was drawn from the AMMP data base using the following criteria: In each household, there had to be a) a woman of thirty to forty years of age, b) who had a child under five and c) had lived in the area for at least five years. To have a woman in the household was, of course, essential for an investigation into health practice and its social organization from a woman's point of view. Since older and younger women might have different conceptions of health and play different roles in the daily organization of health practice, the age range of women in the sample had to be clearly defined and limited. We decided to focus on middle-aged women still involved in raising a small child because such mother-child pairs are often target groups of health programs. The definition of a minimal length of stay aimed to control differences between recent immigrants and more settled urban dwellers.

Of the 2385 households in Ilala Ilala, 129 fulfilled these criteria according to the records. However, we found that some had moved out of the neighborhood or the mother was temporarily absent, others did not meet our criteria because the mother or child had died or because the mother fell out of the age range. 105 households remained. Five of them were selected for the pre-study and 100 for the main sample. The semi-structured interviews with the woman responsible for running the household addressed questions relating to their particular cultural, social and economic background including household structures and headship, their notions of health and health activities, the gender division of responsibilities within and beyond the household and recent illness episodes.

The third component was a study of a cohort of 20 women selected after a preliminary analysis of the household study. These women represented different types of household and headship, aspects we considered as particularly relevant for the investigation of the relationship between gender models and lived gender relations, intra-household divisions and dynamics and participation in wider networks. We visited each of these women every fortnight over a period of three months. During these home visits, we collected data through observation and conversation.

As a fifth component, we conducted focus group discussions with people representing other age and gender categories than our core group of women. The categories comprised younger women (20 to 30 years old), and older women (40 years and older), and men of three age groups (21 to 30 years, 31 to 40 years, 41 years and older). With each category of people, we discussed practices relating to the "water-waste-complex" (Stephens 1996), that is the waster supply system, sanitation and garbage collection.

The last component was classic participant observation. We had the opportunity to rent two rooms in a Swahili house. Living with the people provided many valuable insights into day-to-day health production, its social organization and the flow of life in this neighborhood.

In 2002, the main findings were updated during a field visit. Key informant interviews, informal conversations and observations as well as six focus group discussions with the same gender and age groups as in 1995/1996 were carried out during this follow-up study.

Data analysis was iterative and relied on in-depth interpretation of observational and verbal data, partly using qualitative data analysis programs (Text Base Alpha and MaxQda). To preserve confidentiality, we have changed the names of our respondents.

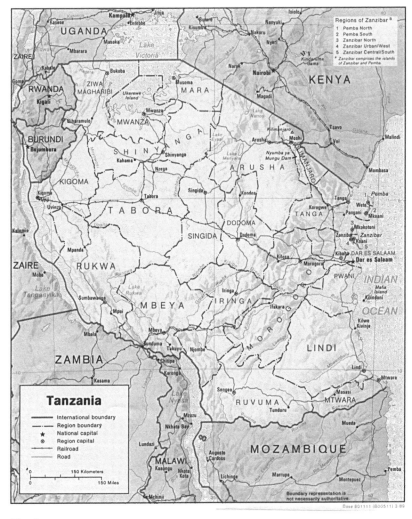

Map 1
Tanzania and the location of Dar es Salaam

70

2 Dynamics and diversity of city life

2.1 Contemporary city life in historical context

Dar es Salaam is a bustling port city on the East African Coast of the Indian Ocean (see Map 1). Although Dodoma has been the official capital of Tanzania since 1973, Dar es Salaam is the industrial, commercial and governmental center. It has a population of nearly 2.5 million (Population and Housing Census 2002). Roads and trains connect the city with distant corners of the countryside, and through its harbor and international airport, Dar es Salaam serves Tanzania and land-locked neighboring countries like Malawi and Zambia as gateway to European, Arabian and Asian countries.

In many ways, Dar es Salaam is just another African city and shares many characteristics with cities in developing countries on other continents: A small commercial center with high-rise buildings, supermarkets and traffic congestion, mushrooming squatter settlements, and more people gaining an income in the informal than in the formal sector. As noted already by Gugler (1988), a certain degree of homogenization of cities has occurred in Africa, whatever their pre-colonial or colonial origin, and between them and cities in other developing countries as they became integrated into the world economic system.

In other respects, Dar es Salaam is anchored in its specific historical, regional and cultural context. Five phases of urban development are of particular interest here. The city was founded as a Swahili settlement and grew into a colonial capital. It then became the center of pride, hope and development in the sovereign state Tanganyika. In the 1980s, it suffered a major crisis, partly due to the worldwide economic recession, partly due to various

71

home-made problems. Under the leadership of the IMF and the World Bank, the national as well as the urban government engaged in fundamental political and economic reforms. Since the mid-1990s, Tanzania and Dar es Salaam have shown signs of gradual recovery. The following sections look at each phase in more detail.

From Swahili town to colonial capital (1862–1960)

As the name indicates, Dar es Salaam (Persian-Arabic: "Haven of Peace") was founded by Persian and Arab traders and belongs to a string of Swahili towns along the East African Coast of the Indian Ocean (Sutton 1970, Köhler 1988, Middleton 1992). Most of the other Swahili towns like Mogadishu, Lamu, Mombasa, Zanzibar and Kilwa, are much older and date back to about 1000 A.D.

While a Swahili culture developed in these old towns through a combination of African, mainly Bantu, traditions and Arabic-Islamic traditions and flourished in the 14th and 15th century, the area of Dar es Salaam remained rural. Only in 1862, Sultan Seyyid Majid of Zanzibar selected this rural site and planned to turn it into the main caravan terminus, port and commercial center of East Africa. However, a few years later he died and his successor was not interested in building the new city.

Dar es Salaam might have disappeared from the map completely had not the Germans decided to make it the capital of *Deutsch-Ostafrika* in 1891. For seventy years, it was a colonial capital and port, first of German East Africa (1884–1914), then of Tanganyika under British administration (1914–1961). Administratively, economically and culturally it thus rose above the local scene.

In other words, the city attained its primacy under colonial rule. The term "urban primacy" refers to the overwhelming economic, social, demographic, and political dominance of the largest city in a country. In Dar es Salaam, as elsewhere, this development is rooted in the colonial economy (Lugalla 1995: 1–18). The largest cities were commonly located on the coast and combined the functions of colonial capital and port. They thus formed gateways between their hinterlands and distant metropoles in the European core countries overseas (Simon 1992: 3).

One can still recognize the colonial division of the city into a "European area" *(Uzunguni)*, an "Asian area" *(Uhindi)* and "African" settlements. The architecture mirrors the colonial history as well as cultural influences from Arabia and Asia. Diverse religious congregations worship in mosques, churches and temples and run schools, hospitals and dispensaries. Already during this first period in city development, Oriental and Occidental traditions became enmeshed with African traditions, creating a new Swahili culture, a Creole culture marked by heterogeneity and diversity.

A period of hope, pride and development (1961–1978)

The second phase began in 1961, when Tanganyika became independent and the late Sir Julius Nyerere[1] her first president. Dar es Salaam turned from a colonial capital to the capital of a sovereign state, a change that had many implications. The government created new training opportunities and comparatively well-paid jobs and built up the harbor, and a number of major industries such as the oil refinery, the aluminum and plastic-ware plant, the cement factory and the new textile mill (Mascarenhas 1967: 45). People flocked to the city in increasing numbers and with high hopes for a better life in the capital of a new society (Teisen 1969: 90). The building of this new society, based on an African version of socialism, has generated much discussion and research within

---

1   Julius Nyerere, one of the most charismatic leaders of 20th century Africa, died in 1999.

and outside the country.[2] Even more importantly, it has shaped the lives of Tanzanians and is deeply ingrained in their personal and social experience.

The vision of an African socialism formulated by Julius Nyerere was based on the principle of *ujamaa* (Swahili for "familyhood") as a starting point of development from below[3].

> The foundation, and the objective, of African socialism is the extended family. The true African socialist does not look on one class of men as his brethren and another as his natural enemies. [...] He rather regards all men as his brethren – as members of his ever extending family. That is why the first article of TANU's creed is: *Binadamu wole ni ndugu zangu, na Africa ni moja.* If this had been originally put in English, it could have been: I believe in Human Brotherhood and the Unity of Africa (Nyerere 1969: 165).

Building on traditional values, especially on equality and co-operation, Nyerere intended to modernize existing structures and to lead his people from equality in poverty towards a higher standard of living (Nyerere 1967: 15, in Trappe 1984: 296). This should be achieved through a rule of social control by TANU (Tanganyika African National Union), the party which had originated in Dar es Salaam and led the independence movement.

In 1964, Tanganyika and Zanzibar merged to form the United Republic of Tanganyika and Zanzibar, an unwieldy name later

---

2   Tanzania is one of the most intensively studied and written about countries of Africa, and the literature produced about it must run into several thousand references (Darch 1996: xv).

3   Trappe (1966) provides a detailed discussion of African socialism with a particular focus on Tanzania. Svendsen and Teisen (1969) give an excellent introduction to the development of Tanzania in the first years of independence with reprints of original documents, and the government publication *Tanzania Today* (1968) captures the spirit of the time. Critical appraisals of this period and the past thirty years by Nyerere and other prominent politicians and scholars have been published by Legum and Mmari (1995).

changed to Tanzania. Tanzania officially became a one-party state under the leadership of TANU. In 1967, TANU adopted a policy on socialism and self-reliance known as the Arusha Declaration in which the idea of *ujamaa* was further developed. The state party and its cellular structure of regions, districts, villages or wards and "ten-house-cells", the policy formulated in the Arusha Declaration and the promotion of Swahili as national language facilitated nation building in a country with about 120 ethnic groups (Omari 1995b). In 1977, TANU merged with a party from Zanzibar to form the CCM *(Chama cha Mapinduzi),* the state party that remained in power until 1992 (Darch 1996). Particularly on the lowest level of administration, local party and state control continued to be closely interrelated well into the 1990s.

In the 1960s and early 1970s, Tanzania made remarkable progress in social and economic development and allocated the majority of her resources to the provision of education, health and other services. Health was seen as an integral part of development, as an asset that would permit people to lead a socially and economically productive life. These and other central values were propagated in nation wide, audio-visual mass communication campaigns propagating slogans like *Uhuru ni Kazi* (Freedom is Work), *Mtu ni Afya* (Man is Health) or *Chakula ni Uhai* (Food is Life).

Of particular interest to this study is the *Mtu ni Afya* health education program that was carefully designed and evaluated in collaboration with foreign experts (Hall 1978). Two million Tanzanians, organized into radio-study groups, followed the twice-weekly broadcasts from May to August 1973, and the title of the campaign soon became part of everyday vocabulary and captured the imagination of many. These broadcasts covered a range of issues in community health, with an emphasis on preventive health. A principal aim of the campaign was "to increase people's awareness of how they can make their lives healthier and to encourage both groups and individuals to take appropriate action" (Hall 1978: 24).

The newly independent government strongly promoted the medicalization of everyday life initiated under colonial rule,[4] and people eagerly participated. Even before the famous WHO/UNICEF conference in Alma Ata embraced the Primary Health Care approach in 1978, health development in Tanzania was oriented towards local communities. Tanzania distinguished itself in this respect.[5] Since the early 1960s, an equitable distribution of health services has been an accepted part of the national development policy.

After signing the Alma Ata Declaration, Tanzania decided to place particular emphasis on the training and use of community health workers to serve the rural areas (Heggenhougen 1986, Heggenhougen et al. 1987). These health policies, radio campaigns as well as the health education offered at schools and health care facilities have, of course, also influenced people's conceptions of health in the city. As we shall see in the next chapter, the Swahili term *afya* (health), originally of Arabic origin, has been attributed new meanings derived from biomedical and public health knowledge.

Tanzania directed most development efforts towards rural areas, where more than 90 percent of the population lived. Like most other developing countries, it underestimated the force of urbanization, a process which had begun to accelerate after the Second World War. In only one decade, the population of Dar es Salaam had nearly doubled, from about 70,000 in 1948 to about 130,000 in 1957. The colonial government tried to stem this tide, but immediately after Independence in 1961, the new state abolished colonial laws and regulations that restricted the flow of

4   The history of health development during German (Koponen 1994, Chapter 7) and British colonial rule (Beck 1981) is well documented and has been critically assessed by Thurshen (1984).

5   As Young (1986: 128) has pointed out, Tanzania was presented as a case study in the influential World Health Organization publication *Health By The People* (Newell 1975) and implicitly held up as a model for other developing countries.

"Africans" into urban areas (Lugalla 1995: 27). Increasing numbers of people migrated to towns and cities, especially to Dar es Salaam (see Table 1).

Table 1
Population growth in Dar es Salaam

Year	Number of inhabitants
1867	ca. 900
1894	10,000
1921	24,600
1948	69,277
1957	128,742
1967	272,821
1978	769,445
1988	1,623,238
2002	2,497,940

Sources: Figures for 1867 to 1957 in Sutton (1970: 19);
Figures from 1967 to 1988 in Lugalla (1995: 21);
Figures for 2002: Population and Housing Census 2002.

The government soon realized that it could not possibly keep step with this rapid urban growth (Lugalla 1995: 161–166). It launched several campaigns to encourage people to stay in their villages unless they had assured employment in the city. When these campaigns did not bring the expected success, the government returned to coercive measures. In 1964, it was declared an offence for unemployed persons to reside in Dar es Salaam. The police began to control people on the streets and those without registered employment were deported to their home areas. Such concerted police efforts were repeated nearly every year, but people continued to return to the city.

Rural-to-urban migration was, of course, not the only factor in rapid urban growth (Kulaba 1989: 208). Natural increase of the urban population and changes in geographical boundaries were contributing factors. In the 1960s and 1970s, the government adopted a number of measures to cope with rapid urban growth (Lugalla 1995: 27–39). It made a major effort, at least on the policy level, to decentralize industrial investments from Dar es Salaam to designated "Growth Pole Centers". It further decided to move the capital from Dar es Salaam to Dodoma, located in the heart of the country, and envisioned Dodoma to become a symbol for socialist ideals, an *Ujamaa* City in a rural setting.

In already existing cities like Dar es Salaam, squatter settlements were rapidly growing due to a shortage of housing. One of the measures taken by the government was to establish a National Housing Corporation (NHC) in 1962 (Lugalla 1995: 50–54). During the first five-year development plan, the NHC built nearly 5000 houses in Dar es Salaam, most of them under the Slum Clearance Program. As will be discussed later, the site of the present study, the neighborhood Ilala Ilala, was completely destroyed and rebuilt under this program (see Chapter 2.3).

The Slum Clearance Program resulted from the president's call to remove old thatched houses in urban areas (Lugalla 1995: 54). The NHC demolished the thatched houses and constructed new houses of "better" quality with materials supplied by the government. The city administration then loaned these houses to the inhabitants (personal communication, National Housing Corporation). In 1969, the national and city administration abolished the Slum Clearance approach because the net increase of housing stock was minimal. New units just replaced old ones. Attention eventually shifted to upgrading squatter settlements.

Foreign consultants supported the Tanzanian government in all these efforts to plan urban development, also in designing the master plans for Dar es Salaam (Heinrich 1987), but rapid urban growth had its own dynamics. In 1967, the urban population accounted for 5.7 percent of the total population of nearly 12 million Tanzanians. A decade later, in 1978, it had reached 13.3 percent of a total population of 17 million (Lugalla 1995: 20).

Even cities in developed countries would have had serious problems to expand infrastructure and services to accommodate such rapid population growth.[6] Cities in developing countries like Tanzania could not possibly live up to this task, and the situation was further exacerbated by the worldwide recession of the late 1970s and early 1980s that hit Tanzania and many other Sub-Saharan African countries particularly hard (Darch 1996).

An urban crisis (1979–1984)

During the third phase, the combined effects of rapid urbanization and economic decline led to much hardship and disappointment in Dar es Salaam. The reasons for economic decline are complex and have caused much debate among national and international experts (Boesen et al. 1986, Svendsen 1995). Today, most authors agree that a combination of external and internal factors have contributed to this decline (Lugalla 1995, Svendsen 1995, Darch 1996).[7]

In the early 1980s, the three typical manifestations of an urban health crisis (see introduction) clearly marked life in Dar es Salaam: 1) a fall of living standards for a majority of urban dwellers, 2) a deterioration of the quality and distribution of basic services, and 3) a decline in the quality of the built and natural environment. We look at each of them in turn.

---

6   I owe this insight to a lecture by Fred W. Krüger, on "Urbanization and Polarization in Developing Countries: Research Activities", held at the Institute of Cultural Geography, Albert-Ludwigs-University of Freiburg i. Br., Germany, on 24 April 1999.

7   Agricultural performance was lower than expected, commitments to public expenditure were high and foreign exchange reserves were nearly depleted. In addition, the economy suffered several unexpected blows in rapid succession. In 1977, the East African Community collapsed. In 1977/78, the coffee boom dropped. From 1978 to 1981, Tanzania fought a war with Uganda. In 1979/80, the oil price doubled. In 1979, there was a flood, in 1979/80 a drought.

Urban residents experienced a much more drastic decline in living standards than peasants did because the consumption of the latter was largely self-provisioned (Bryceson 1990: 191). The real minimum wage in 1983 was at the same level as in 1939, but now it was supposed to cover the needs of an urban nuclear family, not of a bachelor as under British colonial rule. Urban residents faced acute food insecurity (Bryceson 1990: 211) and got accustomed to queuing at shops for staple food purchases.

The government tried to assert its control through various measures. It instituted a party-supervised rationing system (Bryceson 1990: 204) and called on urban councils to allocate farming areas to town dwellers. It launched a campaign called *Nguvu Kazi* (hard work) which legitimated the militia to control men on the street or at home and to send those without valid identification card and proof of employment to a rural area (Bryceson 1990: 209). This affected all unlicensed, self-employed people, including fish sellers, shoe-repairmen and tailors. In Dar es Salaam, the police, national-service soldiers, and people's militia started rounding up thousands of suspected "loiterers" on a random basis.

The government also organized a crackdown on people trying to profit from the scarcities through various black market operations (Svendsen 1995: 120). Tensions increased between the government and people trying to make a living in cities. Men and women were increasingly dissatisfied with a situation in which necessities, from soap to cooking oil, were missing and informal sector activities regarded as loitering (Maliyamkono and Bagachwa 1990).

The deterioration in both the quality and distribution of basic services most obviously included health care and social services, the country's hardest-won achievement. In Dar es Salaam, rapid population growth had outstripped the capacity of the health care system (Lugalla 1995: 97–98) and this, in combination with financial constraints, resulted in poor services due to a lack of equipment, drugs and transportation.[8] Environmental services essential to health, such as water supply and disposal of solid and liquid waste, deteriorated for similar reasons, as the following examples illustrate. The number of urban households grew far more rapidly than the piped water supply system, originally built by the British in the 1950s (Lugalla 1995: 105). Poor maintenance and over-extension led to severe water shortages. Garbage accumulated along the streets. In 1982, thirty-five out of forty-five trucks for garbage collection were out of order due to lack of funds for the purchase of new machinery, maintenance equipment and spare-parts (Kulaba 1989: 223). It was further estimated that, in 1985, less than 10 to 15 percent of Dar es Salaam's population had connection to a central sewerage system (Stren 1989b: 43). At the beginning of the 1990s, a Tanzanian researcher claimed that Dar es Salaam, the former Haven of Peace, was becoming a "garbage and mosquitoes city" (Yhdego 1991: 147).

The decline of the quality of the built and natural urban environment affected people especially in terms of housing. The density of existing settlements increased, as more and more people moved to Dar es Salaam, and previously empty plots became occupied, even in unfavorable physical environments such as swamps or industrial zones. This densification process, however, was not evenly spread out across the city. Partly reflecting colonial divisions, the city's master plans distinguished four types of residential areas (Lugalla 1995: 69):

– Low-Density Residential Areas of high housing standard, located near the Indian Ocean (see Plate 1),
– Medium-Density Residential Areas of medium housing standard, located near the central business district (see Plate 2),

---

8   The situation found in Tanzania, or Dar es Salaam, was not exceptional. According to a study carried out in Côte d'Ivoire, Kenya, Nigeria, Senegal, Sudan, Tanzania and Zaire basic urban services and infrastructure – water supply, garbage removal, road repair, public transportation, health, and educational facilities – were inadequate and in a deteriorating state all across the continent (Stren 1989a: 20).

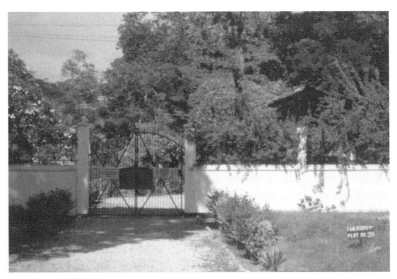

Plate 1
Low-density, high-standard residential area (Photo: B. Obrist van Eeuwijk).

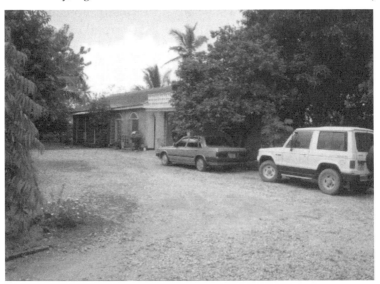

Plate 2
Medium-density, medium-standard residential area (Photo: B. Obrist van Eeuwijk).

82

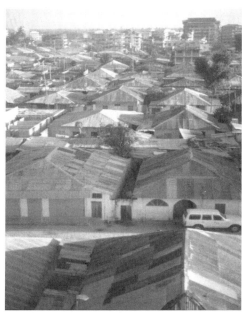

Plate 3
High-density, low-standard
residential area
(Photo: B. Obrist van Eeuwijk).

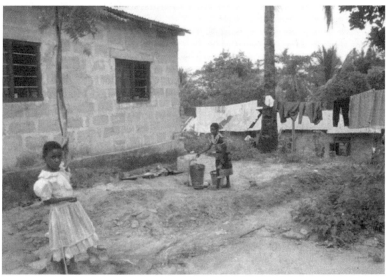

Plate 4
Squatter Settlement (Photo: B. Obrist van Eeuwijk).

83

- High-Density Residential Areas of low housing standard, in the old wards of the city (see Plate 3), and
- Spontaneous Housing or Squatter Settlements of low housing standard, not planned and often not accepted by the government, in disadvantaged areas near the city center or on the periphery (see Plate 4).

In the late 1970s, about 65 percent of the population of Dar es Salaam lived in squatter settlements (Heinrich 1987: 257), and this has not changed much up to now.

It is well known that squatter settlements face problems of overcrowding, inadequate water supply and sanitation, inadequate refuse collection, poor drainage and roads. Squatter settlements are under-serviced and occupied mainly, although not exclusively, by the poor (Lugalla 1995: 43). One often hears the argument that services cannot reach the area because of the irregular layout of these settlements and the absence of infrastructure. What is commonly neglected is that similar problems also exist in planned areas, despite their regular layout and infrastructure, for instance in Kariakoo (Kaitilla 1990). Our study will document this fact for another planned High-Density Residential Area, namely Ilala Ilala.[9]

Even though we focused our discussion on the urban crisis, it is important to bear in mind that the national economic crisis was primarily an agricultural one (Tripp 1997: 62–63). In the 1960s, Tanzania had the highest rate of increase in food production for

9   The Global Report on Human Settlements 2003 assesses and documents the diversity of what is broadly called "slums" (UN-Habitat 2003a). It critically reviews the range of meanings of this term over time and space and discusses controversial explanations of slum formation processes in a globalizing world. From this perspective, the residential area in which the present study was conducted falls into the category of "inner city slum". Although we find it useful to refer to this report in the analysis and interpretation of our data, we do not use the term "slum" because it carries too many – also pejorative – connotations which do not apply to "our" neighborhood.

all of Africa and was exporting food to neighboring countries. By the mid-1970s, the country had to import food, and by the mid-1980s, food accounted for 20 percent of all imports. Moreover, the country's position in the world economy as an exporter of agricultural crops and other primary products set the initial parameters of state capacity. Agricultural products accounted for 80 percent of Tanzania's total export earnings, and these commodities generally suffered from depressed price levels. The agricultural sector, where 85 percent of the population worked, suffered setbacks from the unavailability of foreign and domestic inputs, adequate transportation facilities, and fuel, and this, in turn, led to difficulties in the collection of crops and to crop wastage.

This, at least partly, explains why people continued to migrate to cities, in spite of the urban crisis, and why they stayed there (see Introduction): The root cause of the urban crisis in the 1980s was poverty in its many dimensions whilst inequality within a globalizing economy remains the main challenge, also in the new millennium (UN-Habitat 2003a). Rural poverty drives people to the city and keeps them there, and urban poverty forces them to live under adverse conditions. The result is an "urbanization of poverty".

A period of fundamental reforms (1985–1996)

The year 1985 marked a new beginning for Tanzania. The late Julius Nyerere handed his presidency over to Ali Hassan Mwinyi. This paved the way for an agreement with the IMF and the initiation of a reform process. In 1986, Tanzania embarked on a broad-based Economy Recovery Program supported by the IMF and the World Bank. The new government was called to adjust the exchange rate, to raise official producer prices and to lift price controls (Tripp 1992: 162–163). The donors further demanded that the government improved foreign exchange allocations and made efforts in raising the level of domestic savings, in improvements of the infrastructure and in the launching of major rehabilitation projects. Political leaders also had to introduce measures to which they were initially opposed, such as a fast pace of currency devaluation, constraints on wage increases, and cuts in public services.

The measures were reinforced by an Economic and Social Action Program in 1989 which included a Priority Social Action Program to begin reversing the deterioration of social services that had occurred in the previous decade. The Tanzanian and Swiss governments, for instance, initiated the Dar es Salaam Urban Health Project to improve the health care system of the region. Another example is the Dar es Salaam Sustainable City Program coordinated by the United Nations Center for Human Settlements (UNCHS).

Some reforms were not driven by the IMF, the World Bank and foreign donors but by the collective impact of hundreds of thousands of individuals pursuing similar measures to earn a livelihood (Tripp 1997: 136–141). Struggles over the *Nguvu Kazi* campaign and the legitimacy of self-employment as a means of obtaining a livelihood had been a main tension between those in power and the urban dwellers, including workers and civil servants. By persisting in their informal income-generating activities in defiance of government restrictions, people gradually forced the party officials to shift their policies. In the mid-1980s, open repression of informal sector activities in general gradually gave way to legalization, liberalization, and privatization (Tripp 1997: 136–137).

Political reform began with the introduction of a multi-party system in 1992 after three decades of one-party-rule. The first multiparty elections on the Village, Hamlet and Neighborhood levels *(Mitaa)* were held in 1993. The relationships between the Mwinyi Government and the international group of donors, however, became increasingly strained. Donors were concerned about what they saw as inadequate attention to democratic processes, fiscal mismanagement and corruption (Voipio and Hoebink 1999: 32–33). By the mid-1990s, there was a freeze of foreign aid and, at the same time, great pressure on the government to implement reforms.

Box 1
Newspaper clippings announcing major reforms in Dar es Salaam from July to August 1996.

The Guardian, 13 July 1996: The government broke the monopoly of the National Urban Water Authority (NUWA) by inviting private investors. These investors should start in Dar es Salaam.

The Guardian, 16 July 1996: The Prime Minister dissolved the City Council on 28 June 1996 because it failed to collect enough revenue and to provide the services of which local governments are in charge. A City Commission was installed ad interim.

The Guardian, 17 July 1996: Some politicians of the opposition cautioned against the privatization. One of them asked: "How many of the city residents can afford to buy water from the foreign water companies that have been invited to invest in the sector?"

The Guardian, 17 July 1996: Several factories and companies in Dar es Salaam have closed down in the process of economic reforms. The Gooryong Tanzania Textile Mill, for instance, sacked 1200 workers because it could not raise their salaries from the minimum wage from Tsh 5,000 to Tsh 17,500 as directed by the government.

The Guardian, 19 July 1996: Five companies entered a contract with the Dar es Salaam City Commission to collect the estimated 2,500 tons of solid and liquid waste produced daily in the city.

The Guardian, 23 July 1996: The new City Commission started preparations for a new urban plan to replace the 1979 master plan.

The Guardian, 31 July 1996: As a result of the nation-wide Civil Service Reform Program, 2199 former City Council workers in Dar es Salaam were dismissed in July. Hundreds of them organized a public protest because they had not received the terminal benefits.

The Guardian, 3 August 1996: A simplification of business licensing procedures alone enabled the new City Commission to collect 74.7 million Tsh in one month.

Sunday Observer, 11 August 1996: The move towards privatization of the water sector became necessary because at least 35 to 40 percent of the water pumped by NUWA was lost through leaking water pipes. The water distribution system had outlived its span and had not been rehabilitated.

The Guardian, 14 August 1996: The new procedures led to a crackdown on unlicensed traders in the city.

Sunday Observer, 18 August 1996: The Association of Dar es Salaam Petty Traders (VIBINDO) publicly protested against the demolition of kiosks.

Not only the state, but also the city was in a state of fundamental reorganization. The City Council was dissolved because it did not collect enough revenue and failed to provide public services. The *ad interim* City Commission took drastic measures to collect more money and demolished stalls of street vendors who had not obtained a license. Not only people working in the informal sector but also more than 2000 employees of the City Council were given notice. An even greater number lost their jobs in factories because the employers could not pay them the increased minimum wage. At the same time, the City Council was pushing the privatization of formerly public services, namely of the water supply system and the collection of solid and liquid waste.

The mid-1990s were a very difficult period for the majority of citizens in Dar es Salaam. It was at this time that our ethnographic inquiry into health practice began. People suffered from the manifestations of the urban crisis but also under the rapid reforms which caused much anxiety and social as well as economic insecurity.

For planners, politicians and experts, reforms occur in different sectors. Until recently they have tended to forget that these measures have a cumulative effect on households. Mothers and fathers lose their jobs as civil servants, teachers or factory workers, or they are chased away by City Commission workers as unlicensed traders. At the same time, they are expected to pay (more) for the newly privatized garbage collection services, for health services and school education, and soon an income tax will be collected from them.

For our study, this is a particularly relevant point that has been neglected in previous research. Borrowing an idea put forth by Wilk (1991: 39) in a different context, we argue that the household is the place in the social system where diverse socioeconomic influences and cross-ties come together in a complex knot. Until now, we know little about the ways in which the members of a household try to disentangle this complex knot in day-to-day health practice, particularly in a situation of poverty and rapid urban change.

An era of partial recovery (since 1997)

In its fourth phase, urban development in Dar es Salaam shows signs of gradual recovery. Soon after election, the new president Benjamin Mkapa consolidated the government. Consultations between the government and the donor community improved, and a new agreement was reached with the IMF in November 1996. Since then the national economy has gradually improved, with a GDP growth rate well over 5 percent in the past five years. The Mkapa Government focused on improving fiscal performance and instituting structural reforms. More favorable conditions for investment have been created and attract businessmen from Tanzania and abroad. From 1995 to 2000, the GDP per capita grew by 37 percent (World Bank 2004). The government has increased allocations to social and priority sectors and has implemented a Poverty Reduction Strategy since 2000 (United Republic of Tanzania 2004).

As part of the national decentralization and local government reform program, Dar es Salaam was administratively divided into three municipalities in 2000, based on and named after the previous districts Ilala, Kinondoni and Temeke (Chaligha 2002, Fjeldstad et al. 2003). The City Council, dissolved due to weak management in the mid-1990s, has been reinstalled to coordinate joint activities. To increase popular participation, one councilor from each ward in a municipal area is now elected into the Municipal Council. An important function of these newly formed local governments is the monitoring of formerly public services like water provision and the removal of solid and fluid waste, which have been partly privatized. Many of these improvements have been supported by the Dar es Salaam Urban Health Project and by Dar es Salaam Sustainable City Program. In 2000, these programs were integrated into the newly formed City Council (UN 2001, DUHP 2004).

Several action plans have shown good results (UN-Habitat 2002, DUHP 2004). A private garbage collection system has been introduced. Today, 68 companies employ more than 3000 people;

and there are 17 recycling and composting enterprises. In an effort to keep the city clean *(kuweka jiji safi)*, many women are employed to sweep the streets. A concerted effort was necessary to increase revenue and to enable the municipal councils to deliver services. In the city center, parking areas have been privatized. Street traders now need a license and have been relocated to certain market areas with improved stalls. A fish market and a central bus station have been constructed; those who use the new infrastructure have to pay a fee. In the city center, a one-way-traffic system and the metered street parking have greatly eased traffic congestion. The municipal councils now run all the services and collect taxes. They have formed health boards to streamline the delivery of health care and related services and special security sections for law enforcement. The governmental dispensaries, health centers and the three municipal hospitals under the authority of the City Medical Office of Health have been rehabilitated, the drug supply has been improved and the institutional capacity of the health staff has been strengthened.

In order to tackle the problem of water, the Dar es Salaam Water and Sewerage Authority (DAWASA) was established in 1997 to replace the defunct National Urban Water Authority (NUWA) and later merged with the Dar es Salaam Sewerage and Sanitation Department (DSSD) of the former City Commission (DAWASA 1999–2003). Over the past years, DAWASA licensed many private companies to run water supply and sanitation businesses. Trucks owned by individuals and private companies deliver clean water to city residents, while others empty sewerage tanks, a task formerly monopolized by DAWASA.

In negotiation with the World Bank, DAWASA developed the 61 million US$ Dar es Salaam Water Supply and Sewerage Project. This involves the transformation of DAWASA into a Asset Holding Company sub-contracting the technical and commercial operations to private operators, namely to *Biwater International of UK and Gauff Ingenieure* of Germany, on a 10 year lease (Anonymus 2003).

As elsewhere, privatization, and especially the privatization of water, remains a controversial issue in Tanzania (pers. Communication, Ch. Mayombana). While some worry that private companies have no incentive to provide water to the urban poor, others argue that the poor already pay more than the rich for water. Still others fear that prices for water will surge, when private companies take over the management.

While there clearly have been many improvements on the macro-level and some businesses and people now fare much better than in the 1980s, it has proven difficult to translate structural reforms and economic growth into visible benefits at community and household level (United Republic of Tanzania 2004). Poverty continues to be a primary concern for the majority (TzPPA 2002/03: 59), and most people's living conditions, as observed in the mid-1990s, have hardly changed over the past years. Where changes in city administration and service provision have positively affected households in the study area, we shall of course highlight them. All in all, however, Dar es Salaam residents still refer to their city as *Nchi ya Bongo* ("Bongoland", the place where one always has to use his brains to survive) (TzPPA 2002/03: 161, see also Lugalla 1995: 153).

2.2 The informal sector, gender and social networks

In the 1980s, several social scientists studied people's struggle to gain a livelihood in Dar es Salaam, focusing mainly on squatter settlements.[10] Most of them framed their studies in terms of sur-

10   Mari Aili Tripp (1989, 1992, 1994, 1997) carried out field research in 1987/88, mainly in Manzese and Buguruni. Joe Lugalla (1995) worked at the same time in Kiwalani, Kipawa and Shimo La Udongo. Joachim Mwami (1991) and Felician Tungaraza (1993) conducted their research in the early 1990s, also in Manzese, the largest squatter settlement in Dar es Salaam.

vival strategies (see Chapter 1.5). As their colleagues in other cities, they found that changes in the economy have had an effect on gender relations. The emphasis on men as wage-earners during the colonial time seems to have reinforced local models of gender hierarchy rooted in cultural and religious practice. Since the mid-1950s, urban households have become increasingly organized around men as main breadwinner and authority (Campbell et al. 1995: 222, 243). Women's identity as wives grounded mainly in their responsibility as homemaker and their right and obligation to depend on their husband.

In the 1980s, as a result of the economic crisis, it became increasingly difficult for men to provide for the household (Tripp 1989, 1992). In 1976, husbands' salaries constituted approximately 77 percent of the total household income, in 1988 only 10 percent. This development forced housewives to take up an income generating activity. The percentage of women pursuing such an activity rose from 7 percent in 1971 to 66 percent in 1988.

Tripp (1989, 1992) suggested that women's expanding economic role has given them greater decision making leverage and independence on the household level. Her suggestion generated a lively debate among scholars working in Tanzania (Creighton and Omari 1995). Most other researchers argued that this issue cannot be addressed in general terms and has to be investigated in specific contexts. While Koda (1995) found women's increased involvement in productive work to have both positive and negative effects, Campbell (1995), contended that gender inequality persists and is experienced in two ways. Domestic responsibilities have become redefined, and women have to pursue a variety of activities to generate income. Consequently, women's burden of work and responsibility has increased. In addition, the economic crisis has eroded women's resources, and since men's support is declining, greater demands on limited income and time reinforce female dependence and exacerbate marital relations.

Tripp acknowledged that women's increased involvement in productive work has added to their already heavy workload, but she did not see women as "simply caught between the dictates of a relentless economic situation and the demands of their husbands" (Tripp 1989: 602). She rather allowed for the possibility that women can increase their decision-making leverage and independence, not exclusively but also through acquiring independent sources of income.

This debate continues up to this date (TzPPA 2002/03: 138–139) and provides a context for our analysis of gendered responsibilities in health practice. Focusing on the household, we shall inquire whether women, even if they are constrained by real limitations, can still find ways to take action and to increase their independence and control, or whether the constraints they face reinforce their dependence upon the husband (see Chapter 4).

Researchers working in Dar es Salaam have also shown a concern for social networks (Koda and Omari 1991, Mwami 1991, Tungaraza 1993, Lugalla 1995, Tripp 1997). Some of them took up the concept of "ideology of assistance" formulated by Lomnitz (1977) in her study in Mexico City (Mwami 1991, Lugalla 1995: 90). They asserted that this ideology is dominant in the disadvantaged neighborhoods of Dar es Salaam and works as a reinforcing mechanism of exchange relationships. They further emphasized that people use social networks for many purposes. Members of networks exchange contacts, information and help in the form of money, services, goods or loans. They share facilities and utensils, provide and receive moral and material support or training and apprenticeship, and assist one another in saving small amounts of money. Although people continue to believe in the importance of helping one another, many find it difficult to provide traditional forms of support, for instance from parents to children, husbands to wives and middle aged adults to the elderly, because they are so burdened with their own problems that they have little time or other resources to spare (TzPPA 2002/03: 112). These are clearly signs of social fragmentation, a process which, according to Moser (1998) is a characteristic of urban vulnerability observed in many cities.

People help themselves by defying government regulations, and this has a long tradition. When there was a shortage in water pipes, people dug out underground pipes and sold them (Lugalla 1995: 105). Although the City Council had banned *mikokoteni* (pulled or pushed hand carts) from the city center, people continued to use them as a cheap means of transporting goods (Lugalla 1995: 117). In order to attain goods and services, people went through the "back door" *(mlango wa nyuma)* and "talked well" *(kuzungumza vizuri),* euphemisms for bribing (Lugalla 1995: 122).

Tripp (1997) interpreted people's survival strategies, social networks and involvement in the informal sector as "everyday forms of resistance" (Scott 1985). This concept implies quiet strategies of non-compliance. It differs from popular notions of resistance emphasizing purposeful collective action and organization. Tripp provides many examples of non-compliance and even speaks of a "culture of non-compliance" (Tripp 1997: 179) that developed in the 1980s and conveys a sense of solidarity against state control at its core.[11]

People apply strategies of avoidance, circumvention and advocacy for change up to the present day (TzPPA 2002/03: 74). Several factors, however, limit the effectiveness of these measures, including a lack of voice, poor management of resources and services at the local community level, and corruption.

---

11 This sense of solidarity against state control is well captured in the following anecdote (Tripp (1997: 1): A group of about forty Dar es Salaam passengers had boarded a privately owned *daladala* minibus to go to work. On their way they were stopped by a police officer. At the time this incident occurred in the early 1980s, privately owned buses were illegal. Informal transport had increasingly come into greater use as the needs of the population reached crisis proportions, far exceeding available public services. Realizing they would be in trouble, the passengers, who up until that moment had been perfect strangers, spontaneously transformed themselves into one big, happy family on its way to a wedding and started singing, clapping, and making shrill, ululating sounds, as is the custom for people on their way to celebrations. The police, unable to charge the driver for operating a bus on a commercial basis, had no choice but to let them go.

Most of these studies have concentrated on economic activities to gain a livelihood. What is often neglected is the fact that multiple difficulties also exist in gaining access to services.

> In every item and issue one has to struggle. It is a struggle to get good housing. It is a struggle to secure employment, to get medicine in a public owned hospital, to deposit money in the bank or to withdraw, to get telephone, electricital, or water connection. It is also a battle to board a bus to and from city center, pay the normal official fare, and come back home safely (Lugalla 1995: 118).

Not only gaining a living but also obtaining services has been, and continues to be, a constant struggle in Dar es Salaam, particularly for the poor. In our study, we shall shift the focus from survival strategies to health practice and show that it is also a daily struggle to stay in good health.

Moreover, in previous studies, women, social networks and the informal sector figure more prominently than the household. Creighton and Omari (1995) have noticed the neglect of this important element of the social organization and made first steps to bring some light into local meanings of "household" and its internal organization, but empirical studies from Dar es Salaam are still lacking. Our study will contribute to fill this gap by examining local meanings and household structure in an inner-city neighborhood and by using this construct as focal point of our analysis of everyday health practice.

2.3 Spotlight on an inner-city neighborhood

The site of our research is the inner-city neighborhood Ilala Ilala, about five kilometers from the Central Business District of Dar es Salaam. What is slightly confusing is that the same name "Ilala" is used for administrative units on three levels, namely a branch

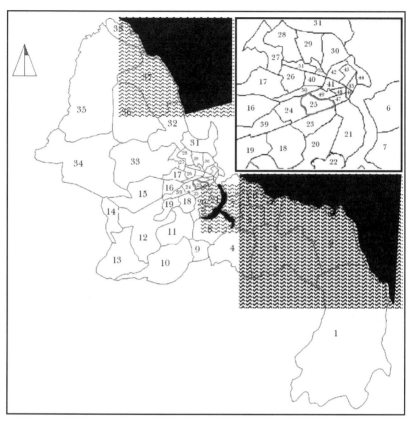

1.	Kimbiji	14.	Pugu	27.	Manzese	40	Mzimuni
2.	Somangira	15.	Kinyerezi	28.	Tandale	41	Jangwani
3.	Kisarawe II	16.	Buguruni	29.	Mwananyamala	42	Upanga West
4.	Toangoma	17.	Mabibo	30.	Kinondoni	43	Upanga East
5.	Kibada	18.	Temeke	31.	Msasani	44	Kivukoni
6.	Kigamboni	19.	Kipawa	32.	Kawe	45	Kisutu
7.	Vijibweni	20.	Miburani	33.	Ubungo	46	Mchafukoge
8.	Mbagala	21.	Kurasini	34.	Kibamba	47	Gerezani
9.	Charambe	22.	Mtoni	35.	Bunju	48	Kariakoo
10.	Yombo Vituka	23.	Keko	36.	Goba	49	Mchikichini
11.	Chamazi	24.	Buguruni	37.	Kunduchi	50	Kigogo
12.	Ukonga	25.	Ilala	38.	Mbweni	51	Ndugumbi
13.	Msongola	26.	Makurumla	39	Vingunguti	52	Magomeni

Map 2
Wards of Dar es Salaam in the mid-1990s (Source DUHP documentation, 1993)

96

(Tawi Ilala), a ward *(Kata Ilala)* and a district *(Wilaya Ilala)* (see Map 3). Moreover, these administrative divisions have been modified in the transformation of the one-part-state into a multi-party-state. We use the term Ilala Ilala to refer to former administrative unit of the *tawi* constituting the neighborhood in which we worked.

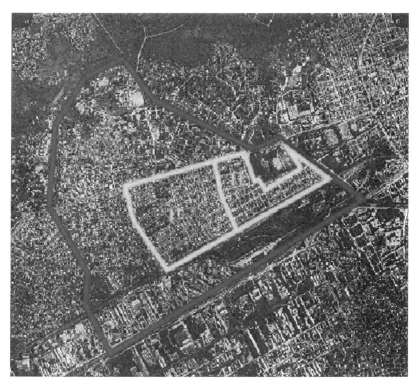

Map 3
Arial photograph of the Ward Ilala with the Tawi Ilala and the Tawi Shaurimoyo (Source: DUHP documentation, 1993)

The British opened the area for settlement in the late 1920s to provide housing for "African workers"; they named it after Ilala in Nyasaland (now Malawi), the homeland of many Yao soldiers recruited by the Germans and the British (Leslie 1963: 22). This has, of course, important implications from an anthropological point of view. The inhabitants of Ilala Ilala do not represent a localized community which has developed shared cultural values and practices over centuries.

In the 1930s, Kariakoo and Ilala were the only "African settlements" of Dar es Salaam. Beyond them, there were only scattered hamlets and single huts. In the mid-1950s, Kariakoo and Ilala were still clearly identifiable settlements, set apart from the city center, the few industrial areas and new African settlements which had developed since the 1920s (Leslie 1963, Map of Dar es Salaam).

After Independence in 1961, the colonial ward Ilala became part of the administrative structure of the one-party state. It was subdivided into branches *(tawi)* and ten-cell-units *(shina)* and integrated into one of three districts of the Dar es Salaam Region. To respond to the shortage of housing, the new government established The National Housing Corporation (NHC). In 1962, the NHC built nearly 5000 houses, most of them under the Slum Clearance Program (Lugalla 1995: 50–54). It demolished the thatched houses and constructed new houses in uniform style with materials supplied by the government. The city administration then loaned these houses to the inhabitants (personal communication, National Housing Corporation).

An old man of Ilala Ilala remembers:

> This area between Shauri Moyo and Bungoni was known as *Bomu* because it was full of trees, not densely settled and considered as dangerous. In 1928, it became one of the main wards under the British. Dwellings of wattle and daub were constructed and covered with palm roofs; they had the same ground plan as now, with a central corridor *(baraza)* and a courtyard *(ua)*. In the early 1960s, the National Housing Corporation started first in Magomeni, then in Ilala. Their representatives came to the houses, took the owners' particulars and asked them whether they wanted to participate. If they said yes, they were told to move out with the furniture. Either a temporary hut was built nearby or they stacked their things with relatives or neighbors. The houses were torn down and rebuilt in about a month. The government fitted everything: electricity, water, sewage chambers, everything.

In the spirit of the 1960s, Ilala Ilala – and other planned residential areas like Kariakoo and Magomeni – was a model of a working class neighborhood in a new urban society. The residents of Ilala Ilala speak of these developments with much pride. They emphasize that the government connected the houses to the city's water supply and electricity system and equipped them with cesspit tanks. Water was available in sufficient quantity and quality, and city trucks passed regularly to collect garbage and to empty cesspit tanks. Even today, one can easily see that Ilala Ilala is a planned settlement. A typical feature is the grid-like layout of streets, dotted with trees and coconut palms (see Plate 5).

Ilala Ilala has a population of nearly 10,000 people (AMMP Data Base 1995). Most residents (60 percent) live in a "Swahili house" (see Plate 6)[12]. These are one-storied buildings covered with some kind of metal sheeting. Each house consists of three rooms on either side of a central corridor that divides the house in half and leads to a courtyard with a communal washing place, toilets and a kitchen. These houses are designed as multi-family houses and commonly used as such. They are the dominant house type in Ilala Ilala. A few wattle and daub constructions still exist; their owners did not join the Slum Clearance Project and currently lack the money or will to invest in reconstruction.

Some Swahili houses have been turned into "contemporary houses" *(nyumba za kisasa)*, usually after they were sold by the original owners. Newcomers and investors employ local construction workers to strengthen the walls with cement, to whitewash, paint or adorn the facades with ornamental stones and to fix iron grids on windows and doors (Plate 7). They install water pumps and flush toilets, rewire the house to ensure connection with the electricity and, if possible, the telephone system. Even more successful and influential residents have built themselves houses with two to four floors *(nyumba za ghorofa)*.

12   These "Swahili" houses do not seem to be traditional of the Swahili villages, rather a twentieth century adaptation (Sutton 1970: 14).

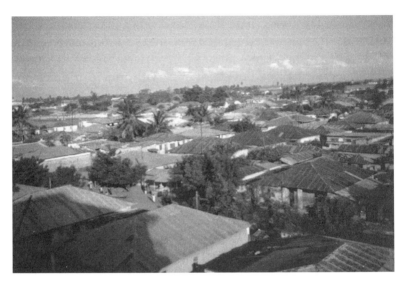

Plate 5
Overview of Ilala Ilala (Photo: B. Obrist van Eeuwijk).

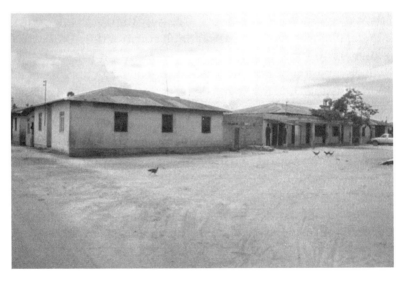

Plate 6
Swahili houses (Photo: B. Obrist van Eeuwijk).

100

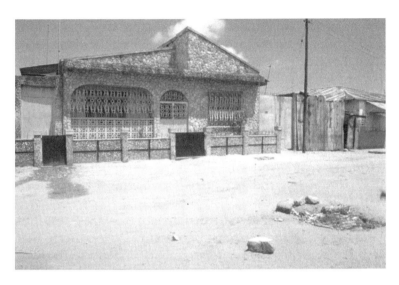

Plate 7
A "contemporary house" (Photo: B. Obrist van Eeuwijk).

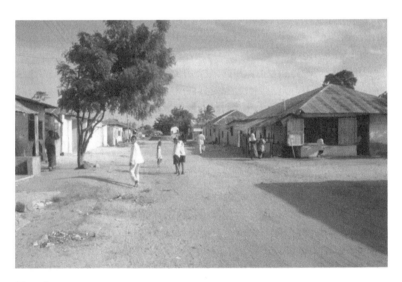

Plate 8
A neighborhood store (Photo: B. Obrist van Eeuwijk).

101

The change of "Swahili houses" to "contemporary houses" and the trend to high-rise structures indicate that Ilala Ilala is again in transition. Located near the expanding Central Business District, the area gradually is becoming a target for real-estate development. Comparatively well-to-do businessmen have bought and reconstructed Swahili houses, using them as one-family-homes. A man of Nyakusa origin, for instance, lives and conducts his business from a two-storied mansion in Ilala Ilala fitted with electricity, telephone and many other amenities. He calls himself "construction contractor" and has bought and renovated fourteen houses that he rents out.

These renovation and construction activities are a result of the liberalization of the Tanzanian economy. They indicate that the gap between richer and poorer segments of the society is widening, not only between but also within residential zones. While a minority can afford "contemporary houses" or multi-storied houses, most people in Ilala Ilala live in dilapidated houses built in the 1960s or even earlier. During the urban crisis of the 1980s, the NHC hardly invested in maintenance. The neighborhood has also suffered from the deterioration of services. As we shall see below in more detail, most government services did not reach the neighborhood in the mid-1990s; and in the last few years, private services have become active (see Chapters 4 and 5).

Ilala Ilala is not only a residential but also a commercial area. Many houses serve as a basis for informal business activities. Some women prepare food and sell it either directly from their homes or from a nearby stall. Others have set up small workshops in or near the house or rent out a space to craftsmen, for instance a tailor or a shoemaker. There are small saloons for hair dressing and cosmetics. Some entrepreneurs have bigger workshops and employ several people, for example carpenters or men specialized in repairing refrigerators, radios or even cars.

There are many shopping facilities. A big, public market with food and non-food sections serves not just this but also adjacent neighborhoods. Scattered throughout the area are more than fifty shops. Some of them are typical Arab and Indian *duka* (see Plate 8) consisting of one room of a Swahili house opened up to the street. Together with the market vendors, they cater for basic household needs such as rice, maize flour, greens and other vegetables, fruit, newspapers, clothes, baskets, brooms, charcoal and plastic or enamel ware. Permanent structures usually require a license, and many women and children sell raw and cooked food from more or less mobile stalls, and men of all ages walk the streets selling anything from coffee to fish or socks.

A number of public and private structures offer services within or near Ilala Ilala. An administrative center of local authorities with a post office and a police station are just across the main street. The district hospital called Amana, the Islamic Dispensary and the Juwata Clinic are in a walking distance of five minutes. After the liberalization of the health sector in 1992/93, a Homoeopathy Health Clinic and two private dispensaries started business in Ilala Ilala staffed with doctors and nurses and equipped with a laboratory. Pharmacies *(maduka ya dawa)* operate in the neighborhood, and a number of ordinary shops *(maduka ya kawaida)* sell medical drugs, for instance Aspirin, Cafenol and Panadol. A few "traditional healers" *(waganga wa kienyeji)* practice in their homes. Right in the center of Ilala Ilala are still other public structures, namely the branch office of the CCM, the Kasulo Primary School, the big Friday mosque and an Anglican church. Restaurants *(hoteli)* and bars offer food, drink and sometimes accommodation.

The market, the shops, health facilities, pharmacies, and the school provide employment in Ilala Ilala, but not all the people who work in Ilala Ilala actually live there. The waiters, barmaids and cooks of bars and restaurants, for instance, come from Buguruni, Bungoni, Magomeni, Sinza, Kigogo, Mtoni and Temeke (see Map 2). Many men and women of Ilala Ilala also work in other parts of the city. They leave the neighborhood early in the morning and return in the afternoon or evening.

2.4 Urban Swahili

Defining the household

Our composite picture of Ilala Ilala residents is mainly based on the study sample of 100 households and complementary data from the AMMP survey (see Chapter 1.7). The AMMP defined the "household" as the group of people who regularly eat together. The concept of "household" however also implies shared residence. In order to clarify, whether only one or both of these aspects are socially relevant in Ilala Ilala, we asked the women in our household study separately about the group of people who live with her in the same house *(nyumba)* or room *(chumba)* and about the group of people who regularly eat "from her pot". In the great majority of households (92 percent), the composition of these two groups was the same. The exceptions include young, single relatives who stayed elsewhere and came to eat in this household. We thus use a definition of the household which is based on shared residence and food consumption.

This does, of course, not mean that the composition of households in Ilala Ilala does not change over time. As reported from other cities, for instance from Lusaka in Zambia (Hansen 1997: 185), people move between households, especially children, adolescents and single women and men, and visits from relatives are frequent. Moreover, due to illness, death or conflicts, households break up and their members rearrange themselves either by setting up new domestic units or by attaching themselves to other households in the same neighborhood or in other parts of the city, and some move out of Dar es Salaam.

Households are not only residential and consumption units, they further have a family basis. Therefore, we asked each woman how the people she lives with are related to her. Based on this criterion, we group the households in our sample into four categories.

Table 2
Household structures (N = 100)

Household types	Total	With foster child	With house helper
Nuclear household	62	18	13
Extended household	20	8	6
Single-parent household	10	3	5
Polygamous household	8	3	2
Total	100	32	26

Since our study was designed to capture the point of view of women fulfilling certain criteria, the sample drawn for the household study (N = 100) does not represent the full range of household structures in this neighborhood. Yet even in this narrowly defined sample, we can distinguish four types of households.

The majority, namely two-thirds of the households, are nuclear in structure. These findings are surprising in view of another study based on the Demographic and Health Survey (DHS) of 1991/92 which suggested that the nuclear family is far from dominant in Dar es Salaam (Omari 1995a: 209–210). According to the DHS, most households (44 percent) comprise three or more related adults, compared to a smaller number of households (38 percent) with two adults of the opposite sex. The seemingly contradictory evidence may be due partly to the difference in sample size, partly to differences in grouping the data. Some of the households we classify as nuclear, for instance, comprise unmarried "children" aged sixteen and older.

It is important to emphasize that we use the term "child" in a classificatory, genealogical sense. Some of these children are young adults, and not all of them were born to the parents they live with. The women or their spouses had them with previous partners, or they were born to brothers, sisters and other relatives of the woman or the spouse. Divorce and changing partnerships are rather common phenomena, not only in Ilala Ilala but also along the Swahili coastal area (Landberg 1986: 113). In the literature, children not born to one of the parents are commonly called foster children.[13] As Table 2 shows, a third of all households comprise foster children. The women themselves made a clear distinction between foster children and house helpers, although both categories consist of adolescent boys and girls, and women take them in for similar reasons.

Our definition of nuclear and extended households differs from that used by Chant (1989) in her overview of urban household structures (see Chapter 1.4). For Chant, extended households are made up of a nuclear family and an attached relative, whether child or adult. Some of the households we classify as "nuclear" would be "extended" in her classification because they include foster children. In our opinion, to subsume nuclear households with foster children and/or house helpers under "extended households" hides more than it reveals.

Extended households, as we define them, have a nuclear core to which adult persons are attached (20 percent). Most extended households in our sample have taken in relatives in need of help, for instance a daughter-in-law and her child, a sick sister, an aged mother or father, or a brother whose family has broken apart, is single or temporarily out of work. Others accommodate non-related persons who work in the family business, for instance in a tailor's shop, a food stall or a shoe store.

The single-parent households in our household study (10 percent) are headed by women who are either widowed, have never been married and/or have a "boyfriend" who hardly supports them. The DHS estimated female-headed households to make up 18 percent of all households, and other surveys indicate a higher percentage of female headed households for urban than rural ar-

13 To raise foster children is a common phenomenon in Tanzania (Omari 1995a) and in many other societies, and one could argue that it is rooted in what Roost Vischer (1997) calls "social parenthood" (soziale Elternschaft). Based on her research in Ouagadougou, Burkina Faso, Roost Vischer (1997: 29) defines "social parenthood" as the distribution of tasks in terms of care and education from infancy to adolescence among relatives of the father and the mother.

eas (Omari 1995a: 215). It is important to keep in mind that our study concentrates on a certain age range, namely women of 30 to 40 years. We would expect that many of the female-headed households in the AMMP sample are young single mothers[14] and older widows raising children.

A household type not discussed by Chant is the polygamous household which makes up 8 percent in our study. In Tanzania, polygamous households are quite numerous, namely 28 percent in the national average (Omari 1995a). They may well be underrepresented in our sample because women mentioned only in passing, if their husband had a second home.

A number of nuclear (N = 11), extended (N = 3), single-parent (N = 2) and polygamous (N = 2) households in our sample live in an arrangement which Chant (1981) calls "compound households". This means that households form separate economic units but have close links with other households in the same Swahili house, either through family ties or friendship. Women commonly referred to this arrangement as living in a or like a "family house". We have not included them in Table 2 because the collaboration between households is an object of investigation in our study and should not be assumed.

Reconstructing ethnicity

In his survey of Dar es Salaam conducted in the mid-1950s, Leslie (1963: 38) reports that the Zaramo, the main "tribe" of this coastal area, made up roughly sixty percent of the inhabitants of Ilala Ilala and about a third of the residents in other settlements. At the end of the 1960s, Vorlaufer (1973: 162) observed that the continuous influx of migrants leads to higher population densities

---

14 Teenage pregnancies are rather frequent in Dar es Salaam and have become recognized as a public health problem (Mpangile et al. 1993, Fuglesang 1997, Obrist van Eeuwijk and Mlangwa 1997).

and ethnic heterogeneity in old neighborhoods. If we define ethnicity in terms of geographical origin and "tribe" *(kabila)*, our data from the mid-1990s confirm the findings of Vorlaufer.[15] The 100 women respondents in our household sample come from 15 out of the 20 mainland regions of Tanzania as well as from the Islands Pemba and Zanzibar (see Appendix I). If the origin of the husbands of married women (N=93) is taken into account, the ethnic heterogeneity is even greater. Most of them come from another region (56 percent) and/or another ethnic group (6 percent) than the wife. All in all, wives and their husbands represent 43 out of the major 120 ethnic groups in Tanzania, and a small group of Indians and Arabs also live in Ilala Ilala. Compared with Leslie's survey, the proportion of Zaramo has greatly decreased, at least according to this sample: Only 13 percent of the women and 11 percent of the men are of Zaramo origin.

In Dar es Salaam, people commonly refer to the residents of Ilala Ilala as Waswahili (Swahili people).[16] What do they mean by this ethnic label? This is a delicate issue because the definition of Swahili identity and ethnicity has been an issue of scholarly and political debate for decades.[17] In its most narrow sense, the

15   Our purposive sample of 100 households is, of course, not representative of the 2385 households in this neighborhood counted by the AMMP (see Chapter 1.7). These are, however, the only data we have because the AMMP did not collect data on ethnic origin.

16   In the Swahili language, prefixes are used to distinguish between the name of the language *(Kiswahili)*, a single member of the Swahili community *(Mswahili)*, the Swahili people *(Waswahili)*, the Swahili culture *(Uswahili)* and the land inhabited by the Swahili *(Uswahilini)*. Mazrui and Shariff (1994: ix) point out that to make this distinction when writing in English "would be to maintain authenticity at the expense of intelligibility". Following these authors, the present study adopts the linguistic rules of the medium of discourse, that is the English language, except for direct quotations of what people say.

17   Many learned articles and books have been published on this issue, and a review of this literature is beyond the scope of this study. Two scholars of Swahili origin, Alamin M. Mazrui and Ibrahim Noor Shariff (1994) provide a thoughtful discussion, and this study follows their usage of the term.

name "Swahili" refers to people originating from the coastal areas. The term Swahili is a derivative of the Arabic *Sawahil*, a word which had multiple meanings in Arabic usage, including coast, coastlands, ports, port-towns and harbors, and the toponym eventually came to refer to the people, their language and their culture (Mazrui and Shariff 1994: 56). Since only half of the women (53 percent) and their husbands (55 percent) in this sample originate from coastal areas, the ethnic label Swahili for Ilala Ilala residents does not quite seem to be justified.

The picture changes, however, if "being a Moslem" is taken as a further marker of Swahili identity (see Plates 9 and 10).

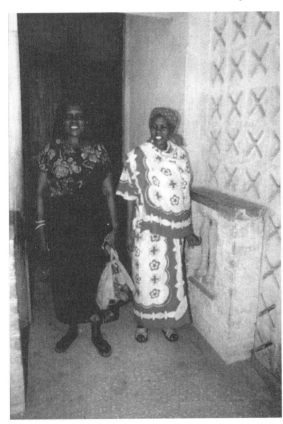

Plate 9
Traditional dress
of Swahili women
(Photo: B. Obrist
van Eeuwijk).

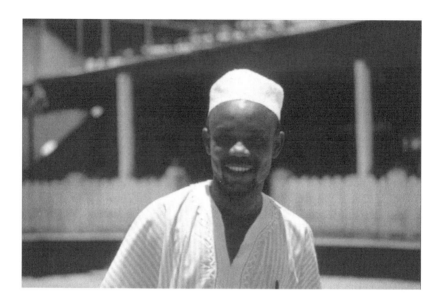

Plate 10
Traditional dress of Swahili men (Photo: B. Obrist van Eeuwijk).

According to Mazrui and Shariff (1994: 34), many East Africans, who adopted the Islamic religion, also took upon themselves the Swahili ethnic label. Whether Islam is a necessary condition for Swahili identity is a controversial issue, even among the Swahili people themselves. Mazrui and Shariff (1994: 34) take the position that it is not Islam as a religion that counts in Swahili identity, but rather Islam as a grid of cultural practices. If affiliation with Islam as religion and/or cultural practice is taken into account, three quarters (73 percent) of the people living in the sample households in Ilala Ilala can be called Swahili (see Table 3).

It must be emphasized, though, that residents of Ilala Ilala do not form a localized, bounded Swahili community socially separated from other localized communities in Dar es Salaam. They share a broader collective identity with people living in other areas of Dar es Salaam, other towns and rural areas of mainland Tanzania, of Zanzibar and Pemba and along the East African coast.

Table 3
Religious affiliation of women and their husbands (N = 93)

Religion	Households		Total (%)
	No.	%	
Moslem			73.0
Unspecified	25	26.9	
Suni	20	21.5	
Ahmadiya	10	10.8	
Shafi	7	7.5	
Ibadhi	4	4.3	
Mixed	2	2.1	
Christian			21.6
Roman Catholic	10	10.8	
Anglican	4	4.3	
Lutheran	1	1.1	
Assembly of God	1	1.1	
Mixed	4	4.3	
Mixed Moslem/Christian	5	5.4	5.4
Total	93	100	100

This is true even if contemporary social organization and cultural practice in Ilala Ilala and probably other parts of Dar es Salaam differ in many ways from those described by Swartz (1991) for the Swahili of Mombasa and by Middleton (1992) for the Swahili of Zanzibar and Lamu. Conceptions of a collective identity called Swahili are dynamic, constructed in time and place and in the context of specific political and economic conditions (Mazrui and Shariff 1994: 53). In our brief outline of the history, we mentioned that Dar es Salaam was founded as the last of a string of Swahili cities in 1862. It was, in other words, not part of the "African mercantile civilization" (Middleton 1992) which had developed much earlier in the other Swahili towns. Since the end of the 19th century until Independence, Dar es Salaam was a colonial capital in which "Africans" from many parts of what is now Tanzania and from other countries were assigned the position of servants, workers or soldiers.

Moreover, conceptions of what constitutes Swahili identity were redefined when Tanzania became an independent state with the goal of building a national identity. Mazrui and Shariff (1994: 45) contend that the socialist policies of Tanzania resulted in a tendency to generalize Swahili identity beyond the boundaries of Swahili ethnicity. The Swahili had to give up their ethnic identity so that it could be turned into public property of the Tanzanian nation. At the same time, the non-Swahili members of Tanzania were required to relinquish their own ethnic identities in order to imbibe a wider and collective identity under a Swahili label. This policy was pursued on terms of the Tanzanian state and not of the Tanzanian people.

The Tanzanian anthropologist and sociologist Omari (1995b: 27–28) presents a slightly different view and argues that the Swahili culture which developed in Dar es Salaam did not belong to any particular ethnic group, and therefore, the Swahili language was well suited as a national idiom. We go even further and suggest that not just the Swahili language and culture built bridges across ethnic and religious divisions and sub-divisions. As outlined earlier, the *ujamaa*-ideology of the one-party-state with its emphasis on "familyhood" and "brotherhood" played an important role as well, and so did the increased geographical mobility and intermingling of people with different ethnic and religious backgrounds, for instance in the villagization program. All these factors contributed to the creation of wider and collective identity, probably more around the verbal symbol of Tanzania than Swahili.

On one hand, we could argue that the majority of the women and men in our study sample share a Swahili culture that developed in the urban setting of Dar es Salaam and is broadly defined by coastal origin and/or Islam as a grid of cultural practices. On the other hand, we have to bear in mind that these women and men have grown up in the newly independent state of Tanzania and have been influenced by its core values transmitted through party and school. They have, at least to a certain extent, developed a collective Tanzanian identity with people who are Christians and/or of other ethnic groups and places of origin.

Collective identities cross-cutting ethnicity

Within this broad Tanzanian identity, we can discern several shared characteristics in our study sample that forge smaller collective identities which cross-cut ethnicity. These are place of upbringing, education, residence and occupation.

In 54 percent of the households both parents, and in 88 percent one of the parents had been born in Dar es Salaam, although not necessarily in Ilala Ilala. They may trace their origin back to diverse ethnic groups and regions, but they have grown up in the same city and lived through the same ups and downs in economic and political development outlined earlier. This social experience has forged a common identity that is not based on ethnicity.

Table 4
Educational level of Ilala Ilala residents

Type of education	Women		Men	
	Household study (%)	AMMP (%)	Household study (%)	AMMP (%)
No formal education	8	12	0	4
Primary education	73	63	56	63
Secondary education	19	25	32	33
Unknown	0	0	12	0
Total	100	100	100	100

Nearly all women and all men have been to school (see Table 4). The majority of the women have primary school education. This means that they have probably been exposed to health education at school. Moreover, they are able to read and write, an important asset in an urban culture. Their spouses are slightly better educated, but even among the women, 20 percent in our sample have a secondary education. The findings of our sample roughly correspond with those of the 1995 house-to-house survey conducted in Ilala Ilala by the AMMP (see Chapter 1.7).

People in Ilala Ilala not only live in a High-Density Settlement, most of them are tenants (72 percent) and live under crowded conditions: In most households (67 percent), four or more persons live in one room (see Table 5). In this case, the figures of the AMMP survey do not correspond with those of our household sample. The higher percentage of one person per room in the AMMP data is probably due to single person households that have not been included in our study sample.

Table 5
Number of persons per room

| Persons per room | Household sample | | AMMP 1995 | |
No.	No.	%	No.	%
1	4	4	4378	47
2–3	29	29	3079	33
4–5	37	37	1040	11
5+	30	30	776	9
Total	100	100	9273	100

In a typical Swahili house built by the National Housing Corporation, all the people dwelling in a house have to share facilities like the sink, the toilet and the shower, which are commonly located in the courtyard. In a house shared by six households with four people per room, this means that twenty-four persons have to use the same facilities.

Concerning occupation, most men (60 percent) are low income wage earners (see Table 6). They work as watchman, clerk, driver, Muslim teacher, accountant, car or railway mechanic, electrician, radio broadcaster, flight plans controller, shoe designer, cashier, soldier, and policeman. A smaller group of men (26 per-

114

cent) are small scale-entrepreneurs and earn a living as tailor, hotel owner, storekeeper, taxi owner, travel operator, carpenter, lorry-driver, fisherman, bus *(daladala)* owner, smith or construction contractor. A third and still smaller group (7 percent) of long distance traders deal with clothes or food between the city and rural areas. One of them traded prawns from Dar es Salaam to Nairobi. Only a few men (4 percent) worked as petty traders, and another small group (3 percent) were retired or recently dismissed.

Table 6
Occupations of men and women

Occupation	Men		Women	
	No.	%	No.	%
Housewife	0	0	31	31
Petty trader	3	4	33	33
Long-distance trader	7	7	5	5
Small.scale entrepreneur	24	26	12	12
Wage-earners	55	60	19	19
Retired	2	2	0	0
Dismissed	1	1	0	0
Total	92[1]	100	100	100

1 Eight women did not have a partner.

It is important to emphasize, however, that the wages of most men are very low. Our data indicate that the situation has not improved since the studies of Tripp (1989, 1992, 1997) in 1987/1988. On the contrary, it is especially the men in the low-level positions who have suffered from the economic reforms outlined earlier. The figures given above reflect the situation in January 1995, and during the following months several men and women in our household sample lost their jobs.

In Tripp's survey in the late 1980s, 66 percent of the women pursued an income-generating activity (Tripp 1992: 165). Our findings in Ilala Ilala are nearly the same: 69 percent of the women are involved in generating income. Most women (50 percent) work in the informal sector. As petty traders (33 percent), they prepare and sell ice cream *(barafu)*, fried fish *(samaki wa kukaanga)*, buns *(maandazi)*, flat bread *(chapati)*, cookies *(kachori)*, rice porridge *(uji wa mchele)* and coffee. Other women deal in cold water, groundnuts, fruit of the baobab tree, mango, coconut, kerosene, wrap-around-cloth *(khanga)* and second-hand clothes. A few women grow vegetables, keep chicken or ducks, embroider, knit or plait mats for sale. Small-scale entrepreneurs (12 percent) work as tailor or traditional healer, own a clothes' shop, a small restaurant, a drug store, a hair saloon, or – together with the husband – a shoe store. Others employ men to tailor, sell water or wash and iron second-hand clothes, and one woman gives tutorials *(masomo ya ziada)*. The long distance traders (5 percent) sell millet or maize from the rural area at a city market, take second-hand clothes to Nairobi and bring back tailoring items, travel to Zambia with music cassettes or buy *khanga* and clothes in Zanzibar and sell them in Dar es Salaam. A rather high number of women (19 percent) are wage-earners. They work as primary school teacher, nurse or nurse attendant, telephone saleswoman, clerk or secretary, cashier, room maid and waitress, and one woman is employed by a Japanese-Tanzanian project to mix and spray anti-mosquito solution.

In terms of employment, the situation has not improved much in Ilala Ilala since the mid-1990s. As in other parts of the city, and indeed in most of Tanzania (TzPAA 2002/03: 69), people mention the problem of employment as a grave concern. Employment opportunities have continuously declined due to a number of factors including retrenchment, freezing of public sector employment and various reforms affecting the parastatal sector.

In terms of residence and men's occupation, the residents of Ilala Ilala can be classified as belonging to the lower ranges of the urban middle-class (see Lugalla 1995: 126–129). They themselves emphasize they are neither *maskini* nor *fukara*, two common Swahili translations of the English term "poor". They point out that many people in Dar es Salaam have an even more difficult life, and refer to disabled persons, street children or beggars as *maskini*. Some men without regular income who often did not know what to eat from one day to the next referred to themselves as *fukara* or *walalohoi*, but they agreed that most people in Ilala Ilala do not fall into this category. They classified them as belonging to a middle category *(kundi la kati)* because they could at least afford to buy food every day and had enough clothes to change them daily.

If we consider collective identities and shared characteristics, we should also bear in mind cultural and social differences. What some people share marks off others, and this creates a web of diversity and heterogeneity. Some people have not been to school while others have primary or even higher education. Some have spent their whole life in Dar es Salaam or Ilala Ilala, others have grown up in a rural area and moved only a few years ago to the city. Some people live crowded in a house occupied by six large households, others share a house with several single person households or have a house of their own. Some men have comparatively well-paid and secure formal sector jobs, others receive a wage that barely covers household expenses for two weeks, and still others draw a comparatively good income from their own business. Moreover, multiple collective identities provide a certain order for social life but also leave space for individuals to define themselves, to develop their own perspectives and to become self-reflective actors.

Gender models

This interplay of collective and personal identity is reflected in gender models. To investigate into this issue, we asked two open-ended questions in our household interview, namely "On whom does your family depend for living?" *(Familia yenu inamtegemea nani kimaisha?)* and "Why?" *(Kwa nini?)*

The women describe four modes of dependence and commonly explain them by identifying with culturally defined gen-

117

der identities and headship (Obrist van Eeuwijk and Minja 1997): The household either depends on 1) the husband, 2) the husband, but with the help of the wife, 3) the parents or 4) the mother.

Table 7
Dependence and headship

	Household depends on…			
	Husband	Husband but…	Parents	Mother
Household type				
Nuclear	41	9	9	3
Extended	13	4	3	–
Single-parent	–	–	2	8
Polygamous	6	1	–	1
Total	60	14	14	12
Women's social characteristics				
Swahili, primary education	45	9	4	6
Swahili, secondary education	7	2	–	1
Non-Swahili, primary education	4	2	7	4
Non-Swahili, secondary education	4	1	3	1
Total	60	14	14	12

As shown in Table 7, gender models reach across household types and social categories based on ethnic and educational background. As in the sample as a whole, Swahili women with primary education dominate in the first and second gender model. However, it should be noted that many Swahili women with secondary education share this view, and so do women of different ethnic and religious background with primary and secondary education. Women embracing the third gender model live in all household types except polygamous households. Even two women heading single-parent households express this view. They have boyfriends who live in the same neighborhood. Women from up-country rather than coastal areas and of Christian rather than of Moslem faith dominate in this third category. Most women of the fourth group head a single-parent household. The three women living in nuclear households explain that the husband is often away because he works as a long-distance trader, is more involved in his work than the home or has retired. The woman in a polygamous household considers herself as the head because she had her children with different men. Half of the women in this group are Swahili, the other half have a different ethnic and religious background. More of these women have a primary than a secondary education.

The first and largest group of women (N = 60) considers the family to depend on the husband *(mume)*. Their explanations vary but center around interrelated themes. Many women say, the husband is the head of household *(kichwa cha nyumba)* and that society gives men this position, whether they work or not. It is the given order, even sanctioned by the Bible.

> He is the one recognized by the society *(anayejulikana)*, even if he does not have his activities, even if he does not work outside. He is recognized as the superior *(mkuu)*.

> God gave every person his/her place. The husband is the head in the house. Even the Bible says so.

> The father is the big one. The husband is the big one. Manhood brings "bigness" *(ukubwa)*.

A related theme is that marriage creates these gender relations. At marriage, the husband takes a woman away from her father and thus has the obligation to provide for her. The marriage gives the wife the right to depend on her husband.

> He took over the responsibility of caring for me [literally "to raise me"] from my father.

> He is the one who married me, who took me away from home. I have the right to depend on him.

Some women link headship with the ability *(uwezo)* of providing for, taking care of and leading the family.

> The superior is the one who leads. I cannot lead. The one who has work is the one who has the say *(ana neno la kusema)* because he is the one who provides food for the family.

> He cares for me. The one who takes care *(mtunzaji)* is the superior *(mkuu)*. He is the one who feeds us, the one who searches for food *(mtafutaji)*. We are just here to cook. I am just the cook *(mpishi)*.

A second group of women (N = 14) first agreed with the first gender model but then had second thoughts which indicate a second, slightly different gender model.

> He is the one who feeds us. He is the breadwinner *(mtafutaji)*. We are just here to cook. It is his honor. Even if I was the one to do it [to provide the daily food]. […] The big ones *(wakuu)* are father and mother.

> My husband is the head. He is the leader of the house. We women have inherited to be led by men. Men are given priority. A woman may have the capability to lead, but because of this inheritance *(urithi)* she leaves the headship to the man. Although a man cannot do anything without being advised by a woman. […] The household is led by the woman. *(Nyumba ni mwanamke)*.

Only a small group of women (N = 14) has a strikingly different understanding of dependence and headship and express a third gender model: They claim their households depend on the parents. These women mention similar criteria as the women in the first two categories, namely the provision of food, care and leadership. What is different is that they emphasize "helping one another" *(kusaidiana)* as an important value of conjugal relationships.

> My husband and I are the heads. The thing is to help one another. He goes to work, and I busy myself with activities at home to generate income. The household depends on both of us. This means that we both are parents. If you look at how difficult life is, one has to collaborate.

A fourth group of women (N = 12) says, their household depends on themselves.

> The household depends on me. I am the one who caters for their needs.

I am the one who is in charge. I have no husband, and I am used to struggling by myself.

At least four interesting points evolve from this discussion. First,
women in Ilala Ilala refer to diverse gender models. This is not
surprising in view of the fact that different and even contradictory gender discourses co-exist in many contemporary societies
(Moore 1994: 824).

Secondly, the social characteristics of the women drawing on
each discourse demonstrate that gender interacts with other axes
of difference, such as ethnicity, religion and education, in ways
which allow for a multiplicity of subject positions within each
discourse (see Moore 1994: 824). Put differently, an individual
woman's stance towards dependence and headship is not determined by particular social characteristics such as ethnicity, religion or education. Women sharing exactly the same characteristics may hold different and even contradictory views, and women
with different social characteristics may share the same view, al-
beit for different reasons.

Third, we found two groups of women saying their household does not depend on a husband as main breadwinner and
authority. One group reports the household to depend on the
parents. As their answers show, this does not mean that they feel
independent or autonomous in relation to their husband. On the
contrary, they speak of "helping one another" which implies
mutual interdependence. The other group of women asserts that
their household depends on themselves. Most of them live in
single-parent households; one cannot say, therefore, that their dependence vis-à-vis their husbands has decreased, but most of them
have become economically and socially independent of the fathers of their children.

The fourth point is that two-thirds of the women describe a
traditional gender model. The husband is the main breadwinner
(*mtafutaji*) and head (*kichwa cha nyumba*), and the wife acts as cook
(*mpishi*) and caretaker of the home (*mtunzaji wa nyumba*). As the

statements indicate, many women take this gender model as a fact of life, some defend it and others look at it critically. Chapter 4 examines, whether these gender models correspond with lived gender relations within households.

2.5 Discussion and conclusions

The terms "dynamics" and "diversity" best capture the contemporary spirit of life in Dar es Salaam. Although the most recent history is marked by a crisis, the 1960s and 1970s were a time of great hope and major achievements and, today, city life implies constraints as well as opportunities for most residents. With regard to the broader forces shaping urban health risks, i.e. environment, economy, governance and society (see Figure 1), our investigation has identified a range of constraining as well as enabling factors shaping people's response options in the study area.

In terms of the environment, there are great disparities in Dar es Salaam, ranging from fully-equipped business centers, hotels and villas forming small islands of gated and carefully tended gardens and parks to ramshackle huts built from scrap material spreading out over vast areas and spilling into industrial zones, swamps and river valleys exposing residents to various natural and man-made hazards. Our research site, the old inner-city neighborhood Ilala Ilala, belongs to the middle range of less privileged residential areas, although it once was a model settlement for low-income workers. Today, the majority of the houses are over-crowded and their infrastructure is run down. Inadequate household water supplies, bad sanitation, insect infestation and accumulation of solid waste in private and public space create a complex of interrelated environmental hazards. However, the area has potential, as some real estate agents and some clever businessmen have realized. Even in its present rather dilapidated state, this neighborhood is better off than many others in Dar es Salaam because of its legal status, its vicinity to the Central Business District and its basic infrastructure in terms of water, electricity and sanitation.

With regard to the economy, we noted a marked difference between the macro- and the micro-perspective. Macroeconomic and related policy reforms adopted since the mid-1980s have helped to reverse some effects of the urban crisis and resulted in overall economic growth. Signs of achievement can be seen in various parts of the city, for instance in new businesses and improved infrastructure. Many of these reforms, however, have had a negative cumulative effect on households, especially among low income workers as represented in our sample. Mothers and fathers lost their jobs as civil servants or employees of parastatal factories but were expected, at the same time, to pay (more) for health services, school education and newly privatized basic services as well as taxes. We argued that until recently policy makers, politicians and experts have tended to overlook that these diverse economic influences and cross-ties come together on the household level resulting in a complex knot.

Economy is closely tied up with governance, and so are the economic and political reforms of the past decades. What we have to bear in mind is that the women in our study, as well as their husbands, grew up and spent their young adulthood during a time of great hope, of political awakening, of building a new society based on the idea of *ujamaa* and African socialism, and then experienced many disappointments and much hardship, both during the actual crisis and the rapid reforms which followed afterwards. This has resulted in quiet strategies of non-compliance, or even a culture of non-compliance, as Tripp (1997) has convincingly argued. An absence of trust in the government, and sometimes even a lack of hope, are sentiments expressed by many, as the Tanzania Participatory Poverty Assessment (2002/03) and ongoing research on the local government reform (Fjeldstad 2004) also document.

123

A hallmark of the Tanzanian society, especially among the Swahili along the East African coast, is a blending of Oriental, African and Occidental traditions, resulting in heterogeneity and diversity. Dar es Salaam is the last of a string of Swahili cities founded along the coast, but due to its late appearance on the scene, it was never a centre of this African mercantile civilization (Middleton 1992). In Dar es Salaam and Tanzania, this blend has been further influenced by Nyerere's attempt to build an African socialist society, emphasizing development through education and labor. This history is reflected in the social identity of our study sample. Most of the participants are of coastal origin and Muslim faith, two common markers of Swahili identity, and belong to the lower ranges of the urban middle-class in the Tanzanian society. But if we look beyond ethnicity, religion and economic status, we find a much more complex situation. What some people share, marks off others, and this creates a web of diversity and flexibility. Some women have not been to school while others have primary or even higher education. Some have spent their whole life in Dar es Salaam or Ilala Ilala, others have grown up in a rural area and moved only a few years ago to the city. Some people live in a crowded house occupied by six large households, others share a house with several single person households or have a house of their own. Some men have comparatively well-paid and secure formal sector jobs, others receive a wage that barely covers household expenses for two weeks, and still others draw a comparatively good income from their own business.

Moreover, multiple collective identities provide a certain order for social life but also leave space for individuals to define themselves, to develop their own perspectives and to become self-reflective actors. Individuals may shift between multiple identities and combine their elements in various ways. This also affects personal gender identity. Women of *diverse* social backgrounds identify themselves with a gender model which defines the husband as main breadwinner and authority. On the other hand, women sharing the *same* characteristics draw on four distinct gen-

124

der models co-existing in the study sample. Still, our data indicate that most women live in a hierarchical gender relationship which is sanctioned by the wider society and defines the husband as superior.

It is within this context of rapid economic and political reforms, social and cultural heterogeneity, diversity and flexibility that everyday health practice in this particular urban neighborhood has to be examined. Daily life in Ilala Ilala is shaped by many opportunities and constraints, and the next chapters will investigate, whether and how individual women in social interactions with others can make use of available options and resist to or even overcome health risks in this urban environment.

3   Everyday health conceptions

We now narrow the focus on everyday health practice in Dar es Salaam and particularly in Ilala Ilala (see Figure 1). When we set out for field research, we knew that *afya,* the common Swahili translation of "health", is used in many different phrases, for instance *huduma za afya* (health care service), *mradi wa afya* (health project) or *kuboresha na kuimarisha hali ya afya* (to improve health conditions). Yet, we did not know what meanings women living in a low-income neighborhood attribute to this term. Do they have a positive notion of health *(afya nzuri),* and if yes, how do they define and explain it? Within which framework do they interpret it, and what do they do for it?

As their colleagues elsewhere, most medical anthropologists in Dar es Salaam (M.-L. Swantz 1986, L. Swantz 1990) and other cities along the Swahili Coast (Swartz 1991, Beckerleg 1994, Schulz-Burgdorf 1994, Swartz 1997, Larsen 1998) have focused on illness, health seeking and healing. Swartz (1991: 225) briefly refers to *afya nzuri* in his discussion of humoral medicine among the Swahili of Mombasa, but his focus is on restoring health in times of illness.

Drawing on previous work of colleagues in Europe (Herzlich 1969, Faltermaier 1994), we elicited local notions of good health *(afya nzuri)* in verbal communication. In our household study, we began the interview by telling women that we would like to learn more about "health in the home" *(afya nyumbani).* After several questions relating to their place of origin, marital status and education, we asked them an open-ended question: "According to your opinion, what is good health?" *(Kwa mawazo yako, afya nzuri ni nini?)* A first group of women (N = 47) formulated their answers in terms of what we have called "health definition" (see Chapter 1.2). They describe signs of good health they observe in themselves but mainly in other people. A second group (N=53) provided "health explanations". They reflect on influences affecting health in their neighborhood.

In order to elicit "health activities", we asked a second open-ended question: "What do you do so that your family is in good health?" *(Utafanya nini ili familia yako iwe na afya nzuri?)* Answers to this question yield information on discursive knowledge or "discursive consciousness" (Giddens 1984: 7). This is of interest by itself because it tells us which activities women regard as beneficial to health. We carried out a content analysis of these verbal accounts in order to identify locally relevant dimensions of "good health".

However, as anthropologists, we are just as much interested in enacted knowledge or "practical consciousness" to follow Giddens. In addition to verbal accounts elicited in an interview situation, we gained insights into local experiences and meanings of health by participating in the daily flow of life, by observing and casually conversing with residents of Ilala Ilala. We draw on these field notes to complement interview data.

The presentation of our data begins with the content analysis. We cut women's responses into segments of recurrent words and phrases and regroup them into categories. We regard the texts we collected not only as a basis for interpretation and an instrument for documenting data but also as an instrument for communicating findings. We shall therefore summarize main findings in the reduced form of tables and then reproduce text passages as evidence for our findings, to illustrate certain points but also to bring certain aspects across to the reader. A disadvantage of this method of presentation is that the flow of reading is interrupted, as one has to follow the rather different logic of different statements. On the other hand, it gives first-hand insights that cannot be conveyed by generalized statements. Since the wording and phrasing of women's answers are of particular importance in such an in-depth analysis, we shall add the Swahili to the English translations. As we move along, we interpret some of the identified meanings in broader contexts and, especially in the section on health activities, increasingly elaborate women's responses to interview questions in conjunction with field notes from our more casual interactions.

On the level of descriptive analysis, the empirical data we present provide a better understanding of health conceptions in this urban neighborhood. On a more analytical level, they can be interpreted with reference to agency and practice. As we present our data, we gradually provide evidence for the development of our argument on both levels of analysis, which we summarize and discuss in the concluding section.

3.1 Health definitions

When we asked women about "good health", they were willing and able to articulate meanings in the form of descriptive definitions and explanations. Many of them found it a rather difficult exercise while others were eager to elaborate on their ideas. In their definitions women identified two main dimensions of good health: the state of the body *(hali ya kimwili)* and the state of the mind *(hali ya kifikira).* To describe each of these dimensions, women refer to several themes (see Table 8).

Table 8
Descriptive definitions of health

Dimensions	Themes
State of the body	Physique
	Appearance
	No sickness
	Functional ability
	Physique
State of the mind	Well-being
	No problems

State of the body

Physique

Women first consider a person's physique *(umbile)* when judging her state of health. An important sign of good health is that the body is portly, round or fattish *(mnene)*, not slim *(hajakonda)*.

> Good health can be seen from the body of a person being portly, not slim. *(Afya nzuri utamwona mtu na mwili wake mnene, hajakonda.)*

Many women share this view, and indeed, it is considered polite to greet a woman by saying "you have gained weight" *(umenenepa)*.

These individual notions draw on cultural values about ideal body shape which differ widely from one society to another, and even within societies, either at a given time or in historical perspective. To have a plump body has been considered as a sign of wealth and general well-being in various parts of Africa and Oceania (Helman 2000: 14), and not long ago also in Europe. Only in the past decades has this body shape become considered as "obesity" and thus as a major health problem, especially in Western countries (Ritenbaugh 1982).

On the other hand, HIV / Aids – a highly stigmatized topic in Tanzania – is often referred to as "slim disease". Although women did not refer to this disease in their interviews, it may well be that this notion has influenced their answers.

Several other women mention body size and shape in combination with body strength, as if they consider both important signs of good health:

> Her body is round, she is not weak, she has strength and is not slim, all right, she has good health. *(Mwili wake ni mnene, hajanyongea, ana nguvunguvu, hajakonda, basi, ana afya nzuri.)*

A third group, however, questions the conventional view that a healthy body has to be fattish. For them "having strength" and "being active" are the decisive indicators.

You look at somebody's body. A person might be fattish but looks weak. Weakness is a sign of illness. *(Unaangalia mwili wa mtu. Anaweza kuwa mnene, lakini anakuwa mnyonge. Unyonge ni dalili ya ugonjwa.)*

Good health is when a person has a strong body, even if she looks slender, as long as she is active, that person has good health. *(Afya nzuri ni mtu kuwa na mwili strong, hata kama ni mwembamba lakini anakuwa active huyo ndiyo mwenye afya nzuri.)*

Even if somebody is slim, but not weak. *(Hata kama ni mwembamba, si mdhaifu.)*

These statements as well as casual conversations and mutual teasing between women and men suggest that "being portly" as a sign of health is becoming increasingly challenged. This may indicate that the currently dominant body image of contemporary Euro-American culture, that is "healthy people are slim and active", is becoming increasingly accepted in Tanzania, also among lower middle class people.

Several women regard the skin as a good indicator for health:

The skin of the person is very important, when you want to check whether one is healthy or not. If the skin of that person looks flabby, then the person does not have good health. *(Ngozi ya mtu ni muhimu sana katika kucheki kama mtu ana afya. Kama ngozi yake imesinyaa, basi, hana afya nzuri.)*

The skin should be soft. *(Ngozi yake iwe laini laini.)*

When you apply oil, it stays. *(Unapopaka mafuta yanakaa.)*

We subsume these statements under the category of "physique" because the skin is both surface and boundary of the body, in a real and symbolic sense.

Appearance

Another set of words and phrases in women's responses also relate to the body, but more to its external appearance *(mwonekano)* than its physique. As the women put it, the appearance should be pleasing *(wa kuridhisha)*, and this means that a person looks well *(anapendeza)*, attractive *(anavutia)*, is "shining" *(amenawiri)*, clean *(safi)* and wears clean clothes *(mavazi safi)*. Some women refer to a "light of the body" *(nuru ya mwili)* or a "light in the face" *(nuru usoni)*. A face which looks dull or pale *(sura imepauka)* is seen as a sign of bad health.

> When a person has good health, you will see that she has a good complexion, looks well, is not dirty. *(Mtu ukiwa na afya nzuri utamwona akanawiri, anapendeza na pia kutokuwa mchafu.)*
>
> Good health can be seen from cleanliness and the face of a person, if it looks dull, you know that her health is not good. *(Afya nzuri unaangalia usafi na sura ya mtu, kama ikiwa imepauka, basi, utajua afya yake siyo nzuri.)*
>
> The cleanliness of a person. When you look at her, you will see a good complexion, and if she is clean, you will not be able to discover whether her health is not good. *(Usafi wa mtu. Ukimtazama utaona ananawiri, na kama msafi, basi, siyo rahisi kugundua kama afya yake siyo nzuri.)*

No sickness

The absence of bodily symptoms of illness is also mentioned by women. They use different phrases like "a person without health problems" *(hana matatizo kiafya)*, "she has no diseases" *(hauna maradhi)*, or "she is not sick now and then" *(haumwi haumwi)*, or:

> Good health means firstly that the family should not be troubled by illnesses. *(Afya nzuri maana yake kwanza familia isisumbuliwe na maradhi.)*
>
> Good health means not to be sick and not to have illness problems. *(Afya nzuri ni kule kutoumwa na kutokuwa na matatizo ya magonjwa.)*

Functional ability

A last set of answers refers to functional ability. This theme is closely related to the idea of strength and the general physical condition, especially when women phrase it in terms of "fitness". At the same time, it adds another dimension, namely being able to do something. This quality is of particular importance to poor people whose body is an important asset for gaining a living.

For adult people this means:

> The body is strong, has strength to be able to do one's business. *(Mwili unakuwa imara, una nguvu za kuweza kufanya shughuli zako.)*
>
> He is fit. *(Yuko fit.)*
>
> To be able to do one's work every day. *(Kuweza kufanya kazi za kila siku.)*

For children it is a sign of health if they play well and eat well. *(Wanacheza vizuri, wanakula vizuri.)*

State of the mind

Well-being

The majority of the terms and phrases women use to describe health concern the state of the body *(hali ya kimwili)*. In a number of statements, however, women mention aspects of health that refer to the state of mind *(hali ya kifikira)*, for instance joy *(furaha)*, wholeness and vitality *(uzima)* or peace in the heart *(amani moyoni)*. A healthy person, they say, is full of life *(mchangamfu)*. We subsume these answers under the category "well-being". As one woman sums it up:

> To be in good health is to be in good condition, physically and mentally. This means vitality, fulfillment of all these things means to be whole. *(Afya nzuri ni kuwa na hali nzuri, kimwili, kifikira. Uzima, utekelezaji wa yote yale ambayo yanafanyika, awe mzima.)*

This statement is particularly interesting because it equates *afya nzuri* with *uzima,* a broader conception of well-being, vitality and wholeness. Several women have used these two concepts as synonyms. These women interpret "health" as an ideal state that goes far beyond the idea of health as absence of disease.

No problems

Others describe "health" in more general terms as "no problems" *(sina matatizo).*

> They do not have small, small problems. *(Hawana matatizo madogo madogo.)*
> He has no problems in life. *(Hana matatizo kimaisha.)*

Such conceptions are nearly as idealistic as "complete well-being" mentioned in the health definition of the WHO quoted earlier (see Chapter 1.1). They certainly express an understanding of health which is based on an underlying idea of a "mindful body" (Scheper-Hughes and Lock 1987), that is a body which is not reduced to its biological dimension.

Similarities and diversity in health definitions

Like similar studies in Europe, we can discern certain patterns in the health definitions formulated by the women in our study sample. The women use both positive and negative definitions of health, often in combinations like "health means a portly body, not a slim one". Their definitions are commonly framed in terms of observable signs, and the women consistently use recurrent words and phrases, which indicates that their personal definitions of health draw on available, collective meanings.

After cutting women's statements into segments in order to identify recurrent themes, we can, in a second step, examine longer statements and see whether and how women combine these elements into multifaceted health definitions. We introduce each statement with the categories we assign to it.

> Well-being, appearance, no sickness
> You look at someone's body. A person in good health is full of life, her clothes are clean, that is she is neat and has no symptoms of sickness. *(Unaangalia body ya mtu. Anaonekana amechangamka, mavazi yake yawe safi, yaani nadhifu bila kuwa na dalili za maradhi.)*

Well-being, physique

You look at a person's condition. If she looks unhappy, weak, not lively, and her body is weak, all right, then she has not a good health condition. (*Unaangalia hali ya mtu. Kama anaonekana hana furaha, mnyonge, siyo mchangamfu, na mwili wake unakuwa umedhoofika, basi, hana afya nzuri.*)

Appearance, no sickness

Good health can be seen from the way a person looks, secondly the clothing, and also not seeing that person suffering from strange illnesses. (*Afya nzuri unaangalia mtu jinsi aonekanavyo na pili mavazi na pia kutomwona mtu na maradhi ya ajabu ajabu.*)

Well-being, functional ability

The eyes of a person, if they are lively, and the way a person walks. Weariness or laziness is a sign of bad health. (*Macho ya mtu kama yamechangamka na jinsi mtu anavyotembea. Ulegevu ni daili ya afya mbaya.*)

No sickness, well-being

Good health means not to have illnesses because when illnesses enter the house, then there will be no understanding. (*Afya nzuri maana yake kusiwe na maradhi kwa sababu maradhi yakishaingia nyumbani basi tena kutakuwa hakuna masikilizano.*)

Appearance, well-being

Good health is the way a person looks, her complexion, and you will see from the face that she is happy. (*Afya nzuri ni jinsi mtu alivyonawiri na utamwona usoni ana furaha.*)

These examples may suffice to illustrate that most women (86 percent) in our study sample mention several aspects of health in their health definitions. Their statements combine aspects of health which – according to our classification – fall into two (52 percent), three (33 percent) or four (2 percent) categories or dimensions. We thus conclude that they formulate not only discrete but also multidimensional definitions of health that draw on collective representations available in the wider society.

3.2 Health explanations

Women's health explanations interweave the two dimensions which we have already identified, i.e. state of the body and state of the mind, with a third dimension, namely "living conditions" *(hali ya maisha)*. The recurring themes we subsume under this dimension are "basic needs", "cleanliness" and "care" (see Table 9).

Table 9
Explanations of health

Dimensions	Themes
State of the body	Physique
	Appearance
	No sickness
	Functional ability
	Physique
State of the mind	Well-being
	No problems
Living conditions	Basic needs
	Cleanliness
	Care

Basic needs

When women talk about basic needs *(mahitaji muhimu)* in relation to health, they mention food *(chakula)*, water *(maji)*, clothing *(mavazi)* and shelter *(nyumba)* – as well as the means to get all of these *(uwezo wa kupata)* – and the environment in which they live *(mazingira)*.

> One should not miss the necessities of life, such as a good house. Also clean water and proper food form part of good health. *(Siyakose mahitaji muhimu katika maisha kama hivi nyumba nzuri. Maji safi na chakula bora pia vinafanya afya nzuri.)*

The children do not sleep hungry. They have clothing. *(Watoto hawalali na njaa, wanavaa.)*

A person living in a good environment is able to get all the basic necessities. *(Anayeishi kwenye mazingira masafi, anapata mahitaji muhimu.)*

Proper food, together with the ability to get the necessities. *(Chakula bora, pamoja na kuwa na uwezo wa kupata mahitaji muhimu.)*

Our study participants used these words and phrases to refer to their concrete life experiences; they reveal the existential health risks some of them are exposed to. It seems that even in this lower middle-class neighborhood some women worry that their children might go hungry.

At the same time, their statements compare with the rhetoric of the basic-needs strategy which became very popular in international organizations including the International Labour Office in the 1970s and 1980s (Trappe 1984: 105). It is well possible that women draw on slogans spread by campaigns to promote a specific strategy or a similar one, for instance in the course of the *ujamaa* movement of the Nyerere Government. That women express their contemporary experience in these words and phrases would then indicate that this rhetoric has turned into a shared and collectively reproduced form of "common sense", similar to the discourse on hygiene and domesticity analyzed by Burke (1996) in Zimbabwe.

Cleanliness

Cleanliness *(usafi)* is another popular concept women often used in their statements. It not only, but also, refers to a clean body and clean clothes, elements already mentioned above under the category "appearance".

Good health in general terms is the cleanliness of one's body, clothes, food and where one lives. *(Afya nzuri kwa nyumba ni usafi wa mwili, mavazi, chakula na mahali mtu anapoishi.)*

It means cleanliness of the house and kitchen utensils. *(Ni usafi wa nyumba pamoja na vyombo.)*

The cleanliness of the pots and dishes, of the rooms inside the house and of the food contribute to good health. Clothes are ironed and clean. *(Usafi wa vyombo, usafi wa ndani pamoja na chakula unachangia afya nzuri. Nguo zinapaswa kuwa safi.)*

The house should have doors and windows for air. Also a clean environment: There should be toilets and a place to put garbage. *(Nyumba iwe na milango na madirisha ya kupitisha hewa vizuri. Usafi wa mazingira: kuwepo na choo, kuwe na sehemu ya kutupia taka.)*

We can, of course, assume that cleanliness has always been a value, both in local traditions and in Islam, but we believe that contemporary notions of cleanliness and health as expressed in these statements draw on a different frame of reference.

In a similar way as food, shelter and clothing have become regarded as "basic needs", cleanliness *(usafi)* has been redefined as a new value within the framework of health development discourses. We would agree that messages disseminated through health education campaigns at clinics and in schools have perhaps not created new conceptual links between cleanliness and health, but we argue that these campaigns have given these concepts new meanings grounded in medical and health sciences, and linked with the idea of development and progress.

This is reflected in phrases like "proper food" *(chakula bora)*, "clean water" *(maji safi)*, "clean environment" *(mazingira safi)* and "cleanliness" in general *(usafi)*. A health education slogan known to many women says: "Without cleanliness, health cannot be achieved." *(Bila usafi afya haipatikani.)* These examples clearly show that the women in our study sample attribute meanings to *afya nzuri* that have been derived from biomedicine and public health.

Care

When talking about "basic needs" and "cleanliness", women often refer to still another concept, namely care *(matunzo)*. Although all these notions are interconnected, "care" often carries a distinct meaning because women use it to emphasize that they take an active role in everyday health practice. The implicit idea is that basic needs do not fulfill themselves and cleanliness does not come about by itself. It is people who work hard to achieve and ensure both. Women speak of

taking care of oneself *(ni kujitunza wewe menyewe)*,

taking care of the children *(kuwatunza watoto)*,

good care of the family *(matunzo mazuri ya familia)*, and

keeping the environment clean *(kutunza mazingira safi)*.

Good care means

making sure the house is clean, washing the dishes and bathing the children *(kuhakikisha usafi wa nyumba, kusafisha vyombo, kuogesha watoto)*,

to clean the environment, the place were you stay and where you sleep *(kufanya usafi wa mazingira yako, sehemu unapokaa na unapolala)*,

to "put the family in cleanliness" is really important if you want your family to be in good health *(kuweka familia katika usafi ndiyo muhimu kama unataka familia iwe na afya nzuri)*.

Other aspects subsumed under the category of care are protective, preventive and curative measures:

to work and rest, to seek medical treatment when your are sick *(ufanye kazi na upumzike, utafute matibabu unapoumwa)*,

hospital services *(huduma za kiafya)*,

now that mosquitoes have multiplied, mosquito nets are important *(mbu wamezidi, vyandarua ni muhimu)*,

to boil drinking water *(kuchemsha maji ya kunywa)*.

These last statements obviously refer to medical care in the Western sense, but local notions of "care" clearly go beyond it.

Similarities and diversity in health explanations

These statements indicate that women construct several links between health and different aspects of their living conditions. First, they link health to the fulfillment of basic needs, particularly food, water, clothing and shelter. Secondly, they associate health with cleanliness or hygiene within and around the home. Third, they emphasize that good care is needed for good health thus indicating a link to the daily conduct of life.

In more general terms, we argue that the women in our study sample construct links between health and social relations, health-related behavior within and around the home, available health services and, in a wider sense, even the urban economy. Their model of "health in the home" *(afya nyumbani)* is similar to the idea captured in the "household production of health" framework discussed earlier (see Chapter 1.4). Women are not only aware of such links, they have a conception of health as something that is not just there but has to be maintained in everyday life through a range of activities. This will become even more obvious in the next section.

If we look at longer segments of women's statements, we find that women formulate explanations centering around the body, the mind and living conditions and combine them in different ways. Each statement refers to shared meanings but differs in detail and represents a personal perspective.

For one woman health means that a person looks clean and infers from a person's appearance to her home. She explains her view by pointing to the link between hygiene and health:

Appearance, no sickness, cleanliness

When a person looks clean. Even if you see her on the road, you will know, her home is not too modest. Many illnesses are a result of dirtiness, therefore good health is in cleanliness. *(Mtu akiwa msafi hata ukimwona njiani utajua kwake si haba. Magonjwa mengi yanatokana na uchafu kwa hiyo afya nzuri iko kwenye usafi.)*

Another woman pays more attention to body shape as a sign of what a person eats and to the skin as an indicator of a clean home:

Physique, basic needs, cleanliness

You look at the person's body and you will be able to know whether she gets three meals or not, or if the person sleeps at a clean place or not. If not, you will see the skin having problems. *(Mtu unamtazama mwili wake ndiyo utajua kama anapata chakula mara tatu au la. Kama analala mahali pasafi au la. Kama si pasafi utaona ngozi yake ina matatizo.)*

A third woman is more critical. She does not judge by appearance or body shape. For her, cleanliness and peace in the home are equally important for good health:

Physique, appearance, cleanliness, well-being

It is not so easy to know what good health is. A person might be portly or smartly dressed, but her place is not clean and peaceful. *(Afya nzuri siyo rahisi kujua ni nini. Mtu anaweza kuwa mnene au akavaa vizuri, lakini kwake hakuna usafi wala amani.)*

What is striking is how many women explicitly mention food, although often in combination with other basic needs, cleanliness or care. This again indicates that for many women having food or being able to eat nutritious food *(chakula bora)* or enough food *(chakula cha kutosha)* is not simply a matter of course.

Basic needs, cleanliness, care

Good health is like that: Children should get food and should not sleep with hunger, they should take their shower properly, and you should also be able to send them to school so that they are educated to know health issues. *(Afya nzuri ndiyo kama hivyo. Watoto wapate kula, wasilale njaa, wakoge vizuri na uweze kuwapeleka shule ili uwape elimu ya kujua mambo ya afya.)*

Basic needs, physique

Good health is the way a person lives, and where she lives and the food she eats; that's what gives a person good condition. *(Afya nzuri ni jinsi mtu anavyoishi na ile sehemu anayoishi na vyakula anvyokula ndiyo vinavyompa mtu hali nzuri.)*

Care, physique

Good health is to know cleanliness and eating well, and this is going to be reflected, when you look at a person's physique. *(Afya nzuri ni kujua usafi na kula vizuri na hii inaonekana ukimtazama mtu maumbile yake.)*

Care, basic needs, appearance

For a person who does not receive care or does not get food you will see even her face looks pale, therefore she cannot have good health. *(Mtu ambaye hana matunzo au hapati chakula utaona hata sura yake imepauka, kwa hiyo hawezi kuwa na afya nzuri.)*

Other women see more complex relationships between food and the state of the body and mind. Eating well is important for good health, but good personal relations and peace are even more relevant:

Basic needs, physique, well-being, appearance

A person may eat well but due to the harassment of her husband she begins to weaken, but the one who is not eating very good food but has a happy time with her husband becomes healthy looking with a bright face. *(Mtu anaweza kula vizuri lakini ananyanyaswa na mume anadhoofika, lakini yule ambaye anakula kauzu lakini anaishi kwa furaha na mume wake ananawiri.)*

Basic needs, well-being, no sickness

Eating well and peacefully forms good health because eating well while there is no peace one might even invite peptic ulcers. *(Kula vizuri na kuishi kwa amani na vizuri kwa sababu kama utakula vizuri bila amani basi utakaribisha hata vidonda vya tumbo.)*

One woman again mentions body strength as a precondition of good health:

Care, physique, basic needs

Good care means that a person should not be weak and should get necessities like food, clothes and a place to sleep. *(Matunzo mazuri yaani mtu asiwe dhaifu na awe anapata yale mahitaji muhimu kama chakula, mavazi na mahali pa kulala.)*

The question of whether a portly or fattish body is a sign – or perhaps also a precondition – of good health comes up again:

> Physique, basic needs, cleanliness, care
>
> Good health is not portliness. Even a slim person can be in good health, if only she gets food, lives in a clean environment and she keeps her body clean. *(Afya nzuri siyo unene. Hata mtu mwembamba anaweza kuwa na afya nzuri ili mradi kama anapata chakula, anaishi pahali pasafi na yeye mwenyewe anatunza usafi wa mwili wake.)*

Some women consider "no sickness" as an important element of health but, as in the case of health definitions, only in combination with other elements:

> No sickness, basic needs, well-being
>
> Good health means firstly that the family should not be troubled by illnesses. Then the family should have necessities starting with food, clothes, shelter, education and peace. *(Afya nzuri maana yake kwanza familia isisumbuliwe na maradhi. Halafu famila iwe na mahitaji ya kutosha kuanzia chakula, nguo, malazi, elimu na amani.)*

As one woman insists, one cannot be healthy without having the financial means to fulfill the basic needs.

> No sickness, basic needs
>
> I see that good health means you, or any other member of the family, should not get ill. If you have enough necessities in your house and especially food, then that is good health. The way I know it, you cannot get good health if you do not have the financial ability. *(Miye naona afya nzuri mtu usiugue wala usiuguliwe na mtu wako. Na kama nyumbani kuna mahitaji ya kutosha hasa chakula, basi, ndiyo afya nzuri. Ninavyojua mimi afya nzuri haiwezi kupatikana kama hamna uwezo.)*

It is just because of these constraints, another woman explains, that one needs to have a "life plan" *(mpangilio na maisha)* which, together with other elements, contributes to good health:

Cleanliness, basic needs, physique, care

Cleanliness and food that builds the body and the life plan in the household bring about good health. *(Usafi na chakula cha kuimarisha mwili na uwe na mpangilio wa maisha ndiyo vinavyoleta afya nzuri.)*

These examples may suffice to highlight ways in which women explain links they see between health and aspects of their daily life. The examples also underline what we have called "agency", namely the capacity to reflect on what one does (see Chapter 1.3). No two statements are the same. Women recur to a range of available ideas, emphasize different elements, weigh the relationships between these elements differently and thus construct their individual views. They are examples of "reflexive monitoring" and of "rationalization" (Giddens 1979: 56). If we had asked the same question again a few days or even months later, women might have emphasized different links or paid more attention to one or another aspect, but we presume their notions would have revolved around the same key categories.

Many of these health explanations express an experience of vulnerability as defined earlier (see Chapter 1.5), namely a sense of exposure in combination with inadequate response options. If we read women's statements as answers to the hypothetical question "what makes people healthy?", we find that having food in sufficient quantity and quality is considered a high priority. This implies the possibility of eating only little or low quality food. Women's emphasis on the fulfillment of basic necessities including food, clothes, shelter, education, a clean home, care and peace also indicate that they do not take these things for granted. To put it differently, women see themselves and their family as being exposed not only to illness but to the risk of not having food and other basic necessities and not being able to fulfill these needs.

This, of course, raises the question what women can do to reduce these health risks. As the subsequent discussion will show, women engage in a range of productive and reproductive activities they consider as beneficial to health. In this sense, they are not defenseless. They describe themselves as reflective actors, who "try hard" *(kujitahidi)* and "make sure" *(kuhakihisha)* to achieve at least minimal standards of nutrition, hygiene and care under difficult circumstances; but they are sadly aware of the fact that their response options are not very effective.

3.3 Health activities

Women's descriptions of health activities elaborate "living conditions", more precisely the themes "basic needs", "cleanliness" and "care" (Table 10). To contextualize our interview data and to highlight certain points, we draw on ethnographic data, partly from our sub-sample (see Appendix 2).

Table 10
Health activities

Categories	Activities
Basic needs	To provide healthy food
	To generate money
Cleanliness	To clean rooms
	To do laundry
	To wash face and body
	To keep home environment clean
	To wash pots and dishes
	To control pests
	To air rooms
	To dispose of garbage
Care	To prevent malaria
	To seek medical care
	To boil drinking water
	To educate children
	To take other preventive measures

Basic needs

To provide healthy food

Daily food provision again comes out as a priority issue. For some women this simply means to have something to eat.

> When there is no illness, the necessary step is to ensure that there is no hunger in the family. *(Kama hakuna maradhi ni kuhakikisha hakuna njaa katika familia.)*
>
> What I do is try to make sure they get food. *(Miye ninachojitahidi ni wapate chakula.)*

For most women the emphasis is more on a healthy diet, on "good food" or "nutritious food" *(chakula kizuri, chakula bora)*, "a mix of different kinds of food" *(vyakula mchanganyiko)*, "to balance the diet" *(kukamilisha mlo)* and to cook "three times a day" *(mara tatu)*.

> First, I make sure that the food for the children is good and enough. *(Kwanza nahakikisha chakula kwa wanangu kizuri na cha kutosha.)*
>
> We should eat good food. Meat, vegetables and fruit should exceed the quantity of maize porridge. *(Tule chakula kizuri. Nyama, mboga na matunda vizidi ugali.)*
>
> I make sure they get different kinds of food. *(Najitahidi wanapata chakula aina mbalimbali.)*
>
> We should get nutritious food, like beans, eggs, and milk, once in a while. *(Tupate chakula bora, maharagwe, mayai, maziwa, siku moja moja.)*

A third group of women puts more emphasis on the cleanliness of food preparation.

> To cook their food in a clean way. *(Kuwapikia chakula kwa usafi.)*
>
> Cooking food in a clean way. *(Kupika chakula kwa usafi.)*
>
> We cover the food. *(Tunafunika chakula.)*

Food and health are closely associated in the minds of most women. They are concerned with feeding the family and, if possible, with preparing quality food in a hygienic way.

To generate money

To feed the family, they need money. In this sense, the generation of income becomes a health activity.

> That is what I have been telling you, we try hard to get money so that we can get the necessities. *(Ndiyo hivyo, tunajitahidi kutafuta pesa, ili tuweze kupata mahitaji muhimu.)*

> To provide for the family needs, for example nutritious food for good health, but financial ability should be there, that means there is no human being who does not like to eat well, but it's hard. *(Kuhudumia familia kimahitaji, mfano chakula bora kwa ajili ya afya nzuri, lakini napo uwezo uwepo, maana hakuna mtu asiyependa kula vizuri, lakini taabu.)*

> You work hard [to earn money], you and your husband help each other. *(Utafanya kazi, unasaidiana na mume wako.)*

> I work hard to get money so that I can buy specific necessities. *(Nafanya kazi kwa bidii ili nipate hela ya kununulia mahitaji maalum.)*

This is a particular feature of the urban environment, where space to grow food is limited. Indeed, many goods that people could produce themselves in rural areas become commodities in the city, including water, food and shelter. For this reason, Moser (1998) has mentioned commoditization as a feature of urban vulnerability. If little money is available to cover a broad range of expenses, some people have to save money on food. Harpham and Molyneux (2001: 122) have pointed out that undernutrition, food insecurity and dietary excess now often exist within the same cities; and these differences are often greater than urban/rural differentials. If, as in our study, people belonging to the low urban middle-class suffer such problems, hunger must be an even more common feature of daily life for many people of the poorer segments of Dar es Salaam society.

Cleanliness

Our study participants went into great detail when they described activities related to cleanliness. For us, these activities may seem too basic or banal to mention, as is the case in food provision, but our study brings to light that it is these very basics that matter most to women in Ilala Ilala. We suggest they matter more to them because they require much effort under the given circumstances. The statement of one woman brings it to the point:

> Keeping the family clean is important, if you want the family to stay healthy. However, what do you do, if there is no water for cleaning? You cannot ask a person about good health, if she has no water. *(Kuweka familia katika usafi ndiyo muhimu kama unataka familia iwe na afya nzuri. Lakini sasa utafanyaje kama hakuna maji ya kufanyia huo usafi? Huwezi kumwuliza mtu mambo ya afya kama hana maji.)*

This is, of course, an exaggeration; people can get water in Ilala Ilala, but the message is that getting water – like getting food – is a daily struggle for most people, and such an environment is not conducive to health. We should bear this in mind as we have a closer look at some health activities subsumed under the heading "cleanliness".

To clean rooms

Many women recount that they sweep, mop, dust, remove cobwebs and change bed sheets. For a thorough cleaning they air the mattresses, wipe out the cupboards and pile everything on the bed to reach every corner.

> I clean the room, I mop the floor, wipe off the dust, and remove cobwebs. I have a day for this. *(Nasafisha nyumba, napiga deki, nafuta vumbi, natoa buibui. Najipangia siku.)*

> I change the bed sheets. *(Nabadilisha mashuka ya vitanda.)*

> I sweep and mop the floor every second day. *(Nafagia na kupiga deki baada ya siku moja.)*

I try to make sure that the place to sleep is clean, the bed sheets, and the bed. *(Najitahidi sehemu ya kulala iwe safi, shuka, kitanda.)*

Each woman follows her own schedule. Some mop every day, others every second day, still others once a week or less often. To consider room cleaning as a health activity makes sense, if we remind ourselves of the crowded living conditions (see Chapter 2.4). In 67 percent of the households in our sample, more than four people share a room.

To do the laundry

Doing the laundry *(kufua nguo)* is another labor-intensive activity, given the environmental conditions. In this hot and humid climate, people change and wash their clothes every day, if they have enough water and soap. The women pour cold water into buckets or plastic basins and soap, rinse and wring the clothes by hand. Washing the clothes for a whole family with this technique is heavy work, and it is even harder, if the water taps run dry and water has to be fetched in other houses or streets, which is the rule rather than the exception in Ilala Ilala.

Not just washing clothes but also ironing them *(kupiga pasi)* is commonly seen as a health activity, not just because it contributes to an attractive appearance, but also because it kills germs. This message is taught in school, and some women have brought it up in the interviews:

To wash dirty clothes and iron them to kill germs bringing illnesses. *(Kuosha nguo chafu na kupasi ili kuwaua wadudu wanaoleta maradhi.)*

Still, not all women share this view as the following notes from a visit in the home of Sakinah illustrate.

Sakinah keeps her own and her children's clothes separate. Asked for the reason she replies this is what health is about. If one member of the family has a skin disease, others will get it from mixing the clothes during the washing. She herself has been suffering from skin disease for a long time. The disease comes and goes. The doctor told her not to share towels with other people and to wash her own clothes separately, if possible. He also advised her to iron her clothes before wearing them and not to wear wet clothes because he thought she suffered from a fungus infection. She has tried out different creams but decided to stop because they did not help. Although she washes the clothes separately, she does not iron them. She explains that since she was born, she has not worn ironed clothes as Europeans do, neither have her children's clothes been ironed up to now, and the children have not suffered any skin disease. Her problem, she asserted, is just like any other disease, it is not caused by not ironing her clothes.

While she complies with the doctor's advice to keep clothes separated in the laundry to prevent the transmission of her skin disease, she does not follow the second part of his advice, namely to iron her clothes. She explains her critical stance by referring to custom and to her own observations, but it is well possible that economic reasons are also involved. Sakinah has to manage with hardly any money because her husband has lost his job as taxi driver, and she herself earns very little by baking buns for a nearby shop. She has no extra money to spend on electricity, even if she owns or has access to an iron. The following passage indicates how precarious her situation is:

A pile of clothes is on the floor, and Sakinah pours water from a rainwater tank into a wide basin. She hands 100 Tsh [1 US$=500 Tsh] to her small son and asks him to buy soap in the shop outside their house. The boy comes back with a small piece of bar soap. She looks at it and asks him who is working at the shop. The boy mentions a name. Sakinah says the size of the bar is too small for the price. She takes it and goes outside. When she comes back, she has a soap of another color. She explains that this brand (Komesha) is good because of its strength. "One piece is enough to do the laundry for the whole house depending on the user."

Sakinah can hardly afford a small piece of soap, and this financial constraint influences her health practice. Many other women are, of course, better off. Those who can afford it prefer washing powder to bar soap because stains dissolve easily without much scrubbing, if clothes have been left to soak for some time.

To wash face and body

Women not only take care of their own cleanliness and take a shower at least once a day, they also take care of the body hygiene of their children.

> We make sure that the children are clean, which means to shower, to wash clothes, to cut nails, to groom hair. *(Usafi wa watoto kucheck, kuoga, kufua, kukata kucha, kusuka.)*

> I make sure that the children wash themselves and brush their teeth. *(Nahakikisha watoto wamenawa na wamepiga mswaki.)*

> We take showers. If it is a child, I wash him or her. *(Tukoge. Kama ni mtoto, ninamkogesha.)*

Bathing babies and small children but also educating older children in body hygiene is seen as an important task of the parents. As Rose, a mother who is also a teacher at the Primary School in Ilala Ilala, explains during one of our visits:

> If I do not remind the children to wash their bodies, they smell because taking a shower is not as important to them as playing. Sometimes they wash themselves without soap, although in school they are told that cleanliness means to wash their body with soap, to brush their teeth, to wash their clothes and to iron them in order to kill the germs. It is not the children's fault at all. Their parents think the teachers are responsible for that, and the teachers do not know whether the children are given any soap at home. A few school children always wear dirty school uniforms, and when they get punished they cry saying there is no soap at home. Some parents bring their children to the teachers' staff room at school for punishment because they do not want to wash their clothes. You should not think all families can afford to keep their children clean.

The school is an important arena for health education, as is the home. Rose insists that parents should enforce hygiene at home but sometimes fail do so, either because they hold the teachers responsible, because they lack the authority or because they do not have the money to buy soap.

To keep the home environment clean

Not just the room and the body, the environment *(mazingira)* should also be kept clean.

> There should be no puddles near the house. *(Kusiwe na dimbwi la maji karibu.)*
>
> We put our environment in a condition of cleanliness. *(Mazingira yetu tunayaweka katika hali ya usafi.)*
>
> The people make sure that the environment is clean. *(Watu wanahakikisha mazingira ni safi.)*

According to our observations, the term *mazingira* in this usage includes the verandah and corridor *(barazani)*, the backyard *(uani)* and, especially if several families share a Swahili house, the communal facilities like the toilet and the shower. Women regularly sweep the verandah and the backyard and clean the toilets with a broom and water. To remove the bad smell, they add ash, cheap soap, kerosene or, if they can afford it, chemical detergents to the water. Others scrub the floor with wastewater from cleaning raw fish or doing the laundry. The subsequent notes were taken during a visit in the home of Grace.

> Grace is busy cleaning the environment. She has a bucket full of water in one hand and a tin of local soap from a nearby industry in the other. According to her, this soap helps to remove the smell in toilets. Some street vendors sell it along the streets. They get it from breweries where the soap is used for washing the bottles. The whole tin is sold at 50 Tsh. When the women buy it, they mix half the tin with ash. Grace distributes the soap all over the toilet floor. Then she adds water and starts to scrub, gradually pouring more water until the bucket is empty.

Each woman has her own method, even if they live in the same house. What "detergent" they use depends on what they consider most effective and can afford.

To wash pots and dishes

To keep the pots and dishes clean is another health activity.

> We wash our dishes and put them out in the sun so that they can dry, and
> then we put them in the cupboard. *(Tuoshe vyombo, tuweke juani kukauka na
> kupanga kabatini.)*

In the backyard of most Swahili houses, there is a big stone sink
(karo) which is used communally and connected to the cesspit.
Women put plastic basins into the *karo,* one for soaping, and another for rinsing. With a small container *(kopo)* they scoop water
from the basins and use coconut husks or plastic sponges to clean
the dishes, and sand or ash to scrub the pots. The *karo* is reserved
for washing laundry, pots and dishes and to bathe babies and
small children. The "*karo* area" and "toilet area" are strictly separated. Women, for instance, scold anyone taking a *kopo* reserved
for the "*karo* area" into the toilet, and they clean the potties in the
toilet.

To control pests

Especially in crowded living conditions, pest control becomes a
health activity.

> I apply insecticide to get rid of cockroaches, rats, bedbugs and fleas. *(Napiga
> dawa kuondoa mende, panya, kunguni, viroboto.)*

> I make sure there are no insects like bedbugs, lice or fleas. *(Nahakikisha
> hakuna wadudu kama kunguni, chawa au viroboto.)*

We have seen many cockroaches, particularly in the "wet zones",
that is in toilets and showers. If people feel bothered and can afford it, they fight them with insecticide but only with limited success. Women frequently complain about pests and take measures
to control them. In many houses, not only cockroaches but also
flies are a big problem, for instance in the home of Sada.

The children sit on the floor having their tea and bread. The breadcrumbs attract flies, and Sada takes out a spray to kill them. Her daughter protests that she always has to cough because of the spray, and Sada laughingly tells her to go outside. She asks us: "What is the best spray against flies? Flies are a big problem in my room, and I find it difficult to control them because we cannot keep the door closed. Particularly rooms towards the backyard are infested because they face the toilets, and the flies bring along the dirt from there."

An even bigger problem for her and many other women are mice and rats, especially during the rain season.

When we come to her house, Sada is busy cleaning her room. She complains about mice. "I have used poison, those black pellets they sell in Kariakoo. We could sleep for about four days, but now there are many more mice than the first time. You know it is difficult to control them because they come from the neighbors. So if two get killed, the week after, four will come into the house. The day after I used the poison in my room, I heard people in the other rooms complain that they have mice. I just laughed."

Each woman has her own story to tell. Some have experimented with cats, others use different kinds of poison or set up traps. A new product called Super Glue is rather popular. It works like glue, if applied on a piece of paper or cardboard. Mice or rats are stuck when they step on it. The women see the advantage of this product in that they can easily locate and kill the animals, whereas poisoned mice and rats tend to hide and are difficult to find until their dead bodies begin to smell.

To air rooms

Another problem for people living under crowded conditions is the lack of fresh air, especially in rooms without windows.

To ensure ventilation. *(Kuhakikisha hewa inapita.)*

To take good care (for instance by ensuring) good ventilation. *(Tupate matunzo mazuri, pumzi safi.)*

154

We have enough windows [to bring in fresh air]. *(Madirisha yawepo ya kutosha.)*

I am building a house, where you have some space, not like this shack here where we are six families. *(Ninajenga nyumba ili kukaa kwa nafasi, siyo kama ninavyo banana hapo, tupo familia sita.)*

We make sure there is a fan. *(Tunahakikisha angalau feni ipo.)*

Our own observations confirm that the air often gets sticky in these houses. This is not only due to crowding. There are few open and green spaces in this neighborhood, except for those around the mosque, the school and the party office. In such a hot and humid climate, trees provide a relief, not only because of the shade they cast but also because they catch and pass on a breeze. One immediately feels the difference, if one visits the low– and middle–density areas, for instance in Oyster Bay. On weekends, people from Ilala Ilala who can afford the transport costs like to go there and capture the sea breeze on one of the public beaches.

To dispose of the garbage

Some women mentioned garbage disposal as a health activity.

We burn or "store" our garbage well. *(Tuchome au kuhifadhi vizuri takataka.)*

There should be a place to put garbage. *(Kuwe na sehemu ya kutupia taka.)*

If I have the means, I volunteer to pay someone to dig a hole for garbage. *(Huwa nikiwa na nafasi najitolea kumlipia mtu ili achimbe shimo la taka.)*

In this house, for example, those people who normally come for garbage, I am the one who pays them. *(Katika nyumba hii, mfano, wale wanaokuja kuchukulia taka, mimi ndiyo nawapa hela.)*

The disposal of garbage is a big problem in Ilala Ilala and has been frequently brought up in day-to-day conversations, during visits in the homes and in focus group discussions. In the mid-1990s, the City Council services had the monopoly but did not collect the garbage; people had to search for alternatives in the informal sector. As these statements show, they either dug holes to bury the garbage or gave it to private collectors. Some people dispose of it at night, as a young woman told us during a focus group discussion:

> We put the garbage in broken pails, and then we take it to a hole at night and throw it away. We do not know whose hole it is. Truly, we do not have a specific place to throw our dirt. *(Tunatia taka kwenye ndoo mbovu, tunaenda kwenye shimo usiku tunatupa, sisi wala hatujui shimo la nani. Kwa kweli hatuna sehemu maalum ya kutupia taka.)*

Only few women mention garbage disposal during the household interviews, probably because we explicitly asked what *they* do for the family health. As we shall see in Chapter 5, garbage disposal is seen as a task of men, not women.

Care

By "care" we mean activities that are closely linked to "basic needs" and "cleanliness" but go beyond, either because they involve a more active role of the people or because they encompass distinct aspects of protective, preventive and curative measures.

To prevent malaria

In the household sample, 21 percent of the women mentioned using mosquito nets.

> At night, we put a mosquito net. *(Usiku tunatumia chandarua.)*
>
> To have mosquito nets to keep away mosquitoes. *(Kuwa na neti kuzuia mbu.)*
>
> I have also mosquito nets. *(Nina neti pia.)*
>
> I put up mosquito nets and wash them once a week. *(Ninaweka vyandarua, navifua mara moja kwa wiki.)*

Several women specify that mosquito nets are particularly important for children. As an alternative, or in addition to bed nets, three women report using coils and sprays.

> To fight the mosquitoes with medicine, with that to burn (coils), if money is little, if there is money, with that to spray. *(Mbu kuwapiga vita kwa dawa, za kuchoma, kama hela ndogo, ikiwepo nanunua za kupuliza.)*

Three women use bed nets and give their children Chloroquine syrup to prevent malaria.

When we visited women at home, they told us how difficult it is to efficiently protect themselves and the children against mosquitoes and malaria. Grace uses a mosquito net as well as coils but still has a problem:

> According to Grace, it is not easy to control mosquitoes in the rooms given the state of the house. "In any house that lacks ceiling boards, mosquitoes move freely from one room to another throughout the night. The malaria shifts from me to my husband and then goes to the children because mosquito coils are no longer effective."

As this statement shows, Grace sees a "mosquito-malaria-link". Her main problem is that even if her family protects itself, they get malaria from mosquitoes that move freely within the house and transmit the disease, presumably from people who do not protect themselves.

Christina relies on coils – and on God.

> Christina tells us that it is difficult to control mosquitoes, especially if the family lives in a single room. Although she admonishes the children to make sure the door is always closed, she normally finds many mosquitoes in the room at night. She uses mosquito coils in the evening, but the mosquitoes become inactive only for a short time, and then they move again. She calls her small daughter and shows us her arms to illustrate how badly mosquitoes bit her since the rains started. Christina, a "born again Christian", then points out that her children have never been admitted to a hospital and attributes this fact to God's power.

Christina is a well-educated woman and knows about the link between mosquitoes and malaria. Like Grace, she questions the effectiveness of coils but still uses them as a protective measure. At the same time, she attributes her children's health primarily to the power of God because she is a deeply religious person.

These findings indicate that women may have a fairly good knowledge of what is good for the health of their family but face many constraints in improving their health practice. These two women are aware of malaria transmission routes[1], but even if they try to protect themselves and their children, their efforts often meet with little success.

To provide medical care

All women mention that, in case of severe sickness, or if small children fall ill, they seek treatment in a health care facility.

> When children are sick, I bring them to the hospital. *(Watoto wakiumwa kuwapeleka hospitali.)*

> When they are sick, I rush them to the hospital so that they can get treatment. *(Wakiumwa, nawahi kuwapeleka hospitali na kuwapatia matibabu.)*

In addition, women say they would seek any kind of treatment, also "home medicine" or "kiosk medicine".

> I search for any kind of medicine, like that of boiling cloves for the stomach. *(Natafuta matibabu mbalimbali, kama vile kuchemsha karafuu kwa tumbo.)*

> If a person has a little bit of fever, I buy drugs. *(Mtu akiwa na homa kidogo namnunulia dawa.)*

As we have seen in the previous chapter, a number of public and private health services operate within or near Ilala Ilala, as well as a number of pharmacies and ordinary shops selling medical drugs (see Chapter 2.3). However, treatment seeking is not con-

---

1   A study on knowledge about the mosquito-malaria link and associated control activities in Ilala and other parts of Dar es Salaam found that people's understanding of the role of a disease vector was high although people had difficulties to distinguish between different types of mosquitoes (Stephens et al. 1995).

fined to Ilala Ilala and its immediate surroundings; people use health care services in other parts of town as well.

> My child Sadam suffered from malaria. We took him to a private hospital, to the Aga Khan hospital in Upanga.

> My child Yusuf had malaria. He was admitted to Burhan hospital in the city center and put on a quinine drip. Burhan hospital serves TANESCO, and this company employs my husband.

Women often visit sick family members or relatives who have been admitted to hospital and bring them food. Relatives from rural areas or other towns are brought to Dar es Salaam, if the illness is considered serious, and this means additional hospital visits for the women. Women also advise each other on home remedies and medical drugs.

> The closer we get to the market, the busier the streets. At one house, Mama Zuhura greets an old man who tells us that his wife is ill. We go into the courtyard, and the woman tells us she suffers from "BP" [blood pressure]. Mama Zuhura advises her to prepare and drink cardamon tea. She asserts this is an old Arab medicine known to help. They talk for a while about how dangerous it is to become dizzy due to BP because it makes you fall and you may hit your head. We say *pole* [condolences offered when somebody suffers] and move on.

> Health and illness are a topic of everyday conversation. People frequently ask about one's health and offer advice. Sometimes they come and ask Mama Zuhura for tablets, specifying the brand names. Mama Zuhura keeps only Panadol at home and buys other medical drugs only when needed, for instance cough syrup, when her granddaughter had a cold.

Some people seek help from various healers *(waganga kienyeji)*, especially if somebody is believed to be bewitched *(kulogwa)*, but "this is hidden, you cannot talk about it, it is your secret" *(utaficha sana, huwezi kusema, ni yako)*. In Ilala Ilala, there are three *waganga wa kienyeji*, two from Tanga and one Zaramo. Many people go to see them as well as healers in other parts of Dar es Salaam, other towns and rural areas.

A man spontaneously explained why some people seek help from healers rather than from hospitals:

> Regarding the problems of sick people, every person follows his environment and his faith (*imani*). For instance, if you have a neighbor, and his child falls ill of *degedege* [a folk illness closely related to cerebral malaria), is brought to the hospital, and is not healed, okay. And you, if your child falls ill of this illness, you might say: "Ah, why was the child of the neighbor brought to the hospital and died?" Okay, you will have the belief that this illness is for the local healer only. And if God agrees to health, all right. Your other neighbor already got the belief that there is nothing else but the healer. Or if you have a brother or a friend who got a headache, was brought to the healer, and was healed, okay. You will also have big faith in the local healer. Some people until now do not have faith in hospitals, until now they very much treasure local medicines.

The explanation of this man is interesting, not only in relation to illness but also to health. It suggests that a person's faith (*imani*) in one or another medical tradition is primarily grounded in personal and social experience, that is in experiences one hears about or observes in a neighbor, relative or friend. Such experiences and reflections also influence people's considerations about protecting health.

To boil drinking water

Several women mentioned the boiling of drinking water as a health activity.

> Water must be clean, we boil it and cover it. (*Maji yawe safi. Tunachemsha na tunafunika.*)

> Drinking water has to be boiled because we do not trust it. (*Maji ya kunywa lazima tuchemshe maana yake hatuna uhakika nayo.*)

> I boil drinking water and put it in a clean vessel. (*Nachemsha maji ya kunywa na naweka kwenye chombo safi.*)

> First, I make sure the drinking water is boiled. (*Kwanza nahakikisha maji ya kunywa yamechemshwa.*)

During the visits in their homes, we found that not all women who actually boil water referred to it during the household interviews. In roughly half of the households in this small sub-sample (see Appendix 2), observation brought to light that people drink boiled water. The other half do not like to be questioned about it and cut their answers rather short:

> I do not boil water for anybody. I believe human beings cannot clean water, but [holy] water can clean them. (Fatuma)

> I do not boil water because the children do not like the taste of it. (Lilian)

> I do not boil water because I am not accustomed to it. (Hadija)

It is difficult to say whether these answers convey deeper convictions or on the spot rationalizations. Still, they are interesting because they illustrate points that are more general. The first statement implicitly refers to the power of God. Similar to Christina, the "born again Christian" who attributes her children's health primarily to the power of God, Fatuma who is a Moslem insinuates that health is not exclusively in the hands of human beings. The second statement alludes to the taste of water. In day-to-day life, people often comment on the taste of water and seem to have clear preferences. The third statement draws attention to custom. People frequently explain their behavior in terms of being or not being accustomed (-zoea) to something. This is one of the reasons why we prefer the concept "practice" to "action"; it carries the connotation of habit.

Other statements show that even women who boil drinking water critically reflect about their practice.

> Amina remarks that she is not sure whether boiling water is really worth the effort. What about the other homes she and her children visit? They may not boil their water, and her family may easily catch diarrhea from them.

> Joyce volunteered that until now she thought boiling drinking water is important, and she makes an effort to prepare safe water for the whole family, not only for the children, as other families do. However, a few days

ago she saw an advertisement for Merry Water on television. In this advertisement – as she understood it – Merry Water was not only praised as cleaner and safer than boiled water, it was also said that Merry Water contains certain bacteria that are useful in maintaining natural immunity when it comes to diarrhea. Joyce says she feels confused because she does not know whether she should continue to boil water and asks for our advice.

Amina's reasoning nicely illustrates a pragmatic stance and, at the same time, makes an implicit reference to the power of custom: It is considered as impolite to reject offers of food and drink. The example of Joyce shows how difficult it is to understand and weigh different bits of information. Both cases draw attention to the fact that women who actively try to improve the health of their families face particular difficulties, for instance because they have to act against custom or because they have only limited access to scientifically correct information.

Those women who are most convinced of the importance of safe drinking water are those who have been affected by a waterborne illness.

Grace is the only one who boils water in this house, and she explains: "I started, when I came out of the hospital, where my second-born was admitted for typhoid; since then I have been boiling water." She admits that it is an expensive habit. One plastic bucket costs 120 Tsh as she has to buy one tin of charcoal. The water lasts only two days because people from other rooms always ask her for drinking water.

The incentive for Grace was that her second-born was admitted for typhoid, and she continues to boil water even under adverse circumstances.

The following account is rather long, but we quote it because it highlights additional aspects.

Victoria is busy preparing safe drinking water. She scrubs a big cooking pot with steel wool and soap, fills it with water from a bucket, puts it on the electric stove and covers it with a lid. While she is doing that, she tells us spontaneously, why she does not trust water from street vendors. One day, she saw one of these vendors fetching water near the brewery. At that particular spot, the used liquids and chemicals from the plant accumulate before they are channeled to an outlet. Since that day, she does not want to buy water from any street vendor. She says "what they care for is their money, not the health of their clients".

By now, the water is boiling. Victoria washes the yellow bucket – reserved for drinking water – and its lid with liquid soap. She explains that she likes the liquid soap so much that she asks the storekeeper at her office for little amounts. She further mentions that, on the weekend, she always boils a lot of drinking water to last the whole week. After she has poured the water into the bucket, she waits until it has cooled down and then fills it into bottles and puts them into her refrigerator.

Victoria tells us, she is very conscious of safe drinking water because she had a bad experience with typhoid. When her little son was one and a half years old, she had to spend a whole month in the Aga Khan Hospital. Never before did she have such stomachaches. Since then, she has not returned to her normal weight and figure. When she was discharged, the doctor advised her to boil drinking water and to carry her own water when traveling. According to her, a person's health is in the person's hands because since then she has not suffered from any stomach problems related to unsafe water. We ask her what kind of stomach problems one could get from unsafe drinking water. She lists frequent diarrhea *(kuharisha ovyoovyo)*, dysentery *(kuhara damu)* and worms *(minyoo)*. She says other people use rainwater for cooking, drinking and other activities, but in her house rainwater was only for mopping floors and washing clothes.

We say other people prefer tap water to boiled water because the latter does not taste good. She agrees that many people do not boil their drinking water and muses about their reasons. Most probably, she suggests, these people have not suffered from serious stomach problems, or if they have, they do not see the cause in contaminated water because they always drank water without boiling it, even when they were healthy. Others, she adds, cannot afford to buy three tins of charcoal a day. They usually buy two tins that cost them 240 Tsh to have their beans and rice or *ugali* [maize] cooked. "Therefore, if you ask them to add one more tin, that is Tsh 120, it means half a kilogram of beans that many people consider enough for a day if one coconut is added. For them, food for the family comes first, not boiled drinking water."

From a methodological point of view, these notes are interesting because they illustrate what participant observation is about. Staying with Victoria in her natural setting brought up the opportunity of observing a practice, and this not only triggered spontaneous information on her part but also opened a space for asking specific questions.

In terms of content, it was interesting to hear that Victoria – like Grace – started to boil water after an episode of typhoid. In her case, she herself fell ill, and she refers to the pain she felt. One could say that her practice of boiling water is grounded in an embodied experience. However, the way she speaks and explains things indicate that there is something beyond this particular experience: Victoria sees herself as a subject of her actions. She herself formulates the idea by saying, "a person's health is in the person's hands". This statement, in fact, not only implies agency but also a moral stance. She has made up her mind how to deal with this problem, and so far her experience has proved her right. When reflecting about people who do not boil their water, she indirectly draws attention to the fact that knowledge and financial means are prerequisites for taking personal responsibility in health matters. For Victoria, in other words, it is "knowledge" *(elimu)* rather than "faith" that counts, together with financial means to put knowledge into practice. We would argue that both concepts, "knowledge" and "faith", can be used as justifications for underlying moral convictions.

To educate children

Many women in Ilala Ilala try to keep an eye on their children, so that they do not play in places that are dangerous to their health.

To restrict the children from playing with dirty water and garbage. But financial means should be there because if you do not want your children to become dirty, then you should at least buy them shoes. *(Kuwanyima watoto wasichezee maji machafu na takataka. Lakini uwezo lazima uwepo kwa sababu kama hutaki watoto wako wachafuke, basi, uwanunulie angalau viatu.)*

I try hard especially for the children. I watch what they eat and what games they play. *(Najitahidi hasa hasa kwa watoto. Naangalia wanachokula na michezo wanayocheza.)*

What I try most is to keep the children and the family well, for instance, that children are not in dangerous places, like playing around water holes or garbage pits. *(Sana sana najitahidi watoto na familia wawe wazima, mfano watoto wasiwe katika hali ya hatari, kucheza kwenye mashimo ya maji na taka.)*

164

During our visits, we found that many women are well aware of their task to educate children in basic hygiene, but they do so with varying success, as the following field notes show:

– Fatuma says she has trouble educating her children on health matters. "They are so dirty, also their clothes. Not one of them likes wearing shoes or slippers. But then, they are all under seven years of age. They are so naughty; I get fed up shouting at them."

– When we arrive, the twins are playing outside, both of them are wearing shoes. We ask Hadija, how she manages to make them wear shoes. "I tell them, if they do not put on their shoes, they are not allowed to play outside, and since they want to go out, they obey." During another visit, she tells us that her elder daughter always makes her bed before leaving for school. She knows how to sweep, mop and cook a meal.

– The small girl Mariamu came from outside and went straight into the toilet with bare feet. Anna says, she feels ashamed seeing her children walking barefoot, especially entering places like the toilet. However, she simply cannot afford shoes for them. Sometimes she instructs them to wash their hands after going to the toilet, but when she remembers that they do not even wear shoes, she just keeps quiet "because what they get via their feet is much worse than what they get from not washing their hands".

– According to Joyce, people in Ilala Ilala can be divided into three categories when it comes to educating children in basic hygiene: Those of the first category try hard because they know the meaning of hygiene and the consequences of not maintaining it. People of the second category try to make their children look like those of the first, but hygiene is not important to them because they trust God to take care of their children. In the third category are those who do not care at all because they think buying second-hand shoes for children is too expensive and because they do not really know about hygiene. She classifies herself as belonging to the first category, and indeed, on many occasions we witness that she makes a great effort to teach her children and constantly worries about their health.

The last statement can be interpreted as a moral judgment. Joyce aligns herself with the first group and dissociates herself with the other two groups. The other statements also tell us something about the values and commitments of each woman, although not explicitly. Fatuma's stance seems to be ambivalent and pragmatic, while Hadija commits herself to educate the children according to her values. Anna reflects about her values and expresses frustration at not being able to live up to them due to financial problems.

A brief look at the background of the four women visited above illustrates that knowledge about hygiene, a sense of responsibility and authority, and financial means interact with one another in complex ways. Fatuma and Hadija have primary school education and are comparatively well situated. Both of them are Moslem, but while Fatuma – as observed on several occasions – tends to let things take their course, Hadija takes them into her own hands. Anna is a single parent and was rather well off when we first met her, but at the time of this visit, her luck had dramatically changed: She had lost her job as secretary and hardly knew how to obtain food from one day to the next. Joyce, like Anna, is a Christian and has higher education. She was well off during our first meetings but then faced growing financial problems as her husband stayed away longer than planned on a business trip to South Africa. First Anna and later Joyce became increasingly frustrated because they had to direct most of their efforts at getting food and had little time, energy and money left for educating their children in hygiene.

To take other preventive measures

A few women in our sample mention a medical checkup or seeking advice from the doctor.

To check the children at the hospital now and then, for instance whether they have worms. *(Kuwapima watoto mara kwa mara, minyoo.)*

I keep an eye on all the things mentioned above. If I see I cannot fulfill them and fail, I go to see a doctor. *(Nitaangalia hivyo vilivyotajwa hapo juu. Nikiona sijavitekeleza na ninashindwa nitaenda kwa daktari.)*

We also included "praying" in this category because it means that people recur to a higher authority in order to avert affliction. As one woman put it:

Even more, we live in the trust of prayers. I may be shown [I may dream] that my child is sick, so I pray for the spirit of sickness to get broken, to get away from us. At another time, we may be shown that a car knocks down the child, so we pray against the spirit of death. Therefore, prayers are our pillars. *(Zaidi tunaishi ndani maombi. Naweza kuonyeshwa mtoto ni mgonjwa kwa hiyo tunaomba pepo la maradhi livunjike, tuepukane nalo. Saa nyingine, tunaonyeshwa mtoto akagongwa na gari, tunakemea pepo la mauti.)*

It is important to bear in mind that the frequency of spontaneous mentioning is a poor indicator of actual practice. We can assume that few women can afford a medical checkup for their children, but many seek advice, although not only from doctors but also from anyone they know who might offer an informed opinion. The idea to seek protection and to avert sickness is not new. Many people visit healers to ask for prayers and protection.

There are protections of many kinds. *Kinga* is a medicine you receive from a local healer or you find it yourself in order to protect yourself against any kind of bad thing, like being bewitched, or being followed by spirits. The healer makes you a charm and tells you, you should wear it on the neck, the hand, the hip or to put it in the pocket and to walk with it every-where you go, so that it protects you from these bad things.

Women in Ilala Ilala, in other words, seek the help of various authorities and powers for the prevention of sickness and the protection of their own and their family's health. To whom they turn depends on various factors including the problem or purpose at hand, their moral stance and their financial means.

Similarities and diversity in health activities

As in the case of health definitions and health explanations, we find that women's statements combine these elements in many different ways drawing on a set of shared ideas. To give a few examples:

> I do a lot of small trade so that I can buy green vegetables. I buy mosquito coils for my children. I search for any kind of medicine, like that of boiling cloves for the stomach. *(Nafanya vibiashara vingi vingi angalau tuweze kununua mboga. Huwa nawanunulia watoto dawa ya mbu ya kuchoma. Kutafuta matibabu mbalimbali kama vile kuchemsha karafuu kwa tumbo.)*

> The first thing is to make sure the family does not get malaria. I normally give the children Chloroquine syrup once a week. Secondly, I make sure that the children get medical drugs when they have a fever, together with proper food. *(Kwanza ni kuhakikisha familia haipati malaria. Huwa nawapa watoto Chloroquine syrup mara moja kwa wiki. Pili, kuhakikisha wanapata dawa wanapokuwa na homa na chakula kinachofaa.)*

> I boil drinking water, care for nutrition and look after the sick when they fall ill. *(Nachemsha maji ya kunywa, najali lishe na nashughulikia wagonjwa wanapokuwa wanaumwa).*

Even though the statements of individual women differ, they center around five main types of health activities. Women try hard to feed the family members and, if possible, to cook balanced meals in a hygienic way. Much of their time and energy goes into personal and home hygiene, and this includes getting water in sufficient quantity for mopping floors, doing the laundry, taking showers and washing dishes. Looking after small children is another principal concern of the women. They further take care of and visit sick family members and relatives. Last but not least, they contribute to household income in order to fulfill these basic needs.

3.4 Discussion and conclusions

In this chapter we examined health conceptions as a response option to urban health risks on the individual and household levels (see Figure 1). The central question was whether women in this inner-city neighborhood of Dar es Salaam have access to, and command of, health knowledge that enables them to respond in a socially accepted and effective way to urban health risks. In a first step, and building on previous research in Europe (Faltermaier 1994, Faltermaier et al. 1998), we investigated local health conceptions, i.e. what "good health" actually means to these women and what they do for it in everyday life. In a second step, we reconsidered these health conceptions in terms of "agency" and "practice" and analyzed whether and how individual women put them to good use.

On a first, descriptive level of analysis, we find that women in our study are able to formulate not only discrete but multidimensional concepts of good health *(afya nzuri)* that draw on collective representations available in the wider society. In their descriptive health definitions, women first consider the condition of the body *(hali ya kimwili)*, whether it is portly, strong and looking well, and then the condition of the mind *(hali ya kifikira)*, looking for signs like joy, vitality and peace. Their health explanations link conditions of the body and mind with specific living conditions *(hali ya maisha)*, emphasizing basic needs, cleanliness and care. When women describe health activities, they also refer to urban living conditions and specify five main themes: 1) to generate income, 2) to provide nutritious food, 3) to ensure cleanliness, 4) to take care of children, and 5) to provide health care.

These meanings of health document that women in Ilala Ilala construct several links between health and aspects of urban life. First, they see the fulfillment of basic needs, particularly food, water, clothing and shelter, as a prerequisite for health. Secondly, they consider cleanliness or hygiene within and around the home as essential for good health. And third, they emphasize that good care is needed for good health, thus indicating a link with the daily conduct of life. In more general terms, we argue that these women link health with basic necessities and hygiene within and around the home, self care and care of significant others, health and other basic services and, in a wider sense, the urban environment, economy, government and society. Their model of "health in the home" *(afya nyumbani)* is similar to the idea captured in the "household production of health" framework discussed earlier (see Chapter 1.4). Moreover, women are not only aware of linkage between health and urban risks, they have a conception of health as something that is not just there but has to be maintained in everyday life through a range of productive and reproductive activities. This will become even clearer in the next chapters.

On a second, more analytical level we claim that these health conceptions refer to real life experiences as well as to existing frameworks for interpreting these experiences. Even in this lower middle-class neighborhood, some women in our study are confronted with very real, existential health risks: They worry that their children might go hungry. Not just for these but for most women in Ilala Ilala food and health are closely associated, and one of their main concerns is to feed the family regularly and adequately. This finding confirms that food insecurity is not just a rural phenomenon (Harpham and Molyneux 2001: 122).

As women try to make sense of their personal experience, they draw on and combine frameworks representing social experience. These frameworks are products of history and of ongoing debates in public and private arenas and are fed by diverse traditions, sources and media. The notion of "good health" presented above is a composite influenced by several frameworks. Ideas like *uzima* (vitality, life force) and *amani* (peace) refer to broader understandings of health and well-being in Bantu as well as Christian and Islamic religious thought. However, understandings of *afya nzuri* drawing on a framework of humoral notions rooted in Arabic medicine as reported by Swartz (1991) for Mombasa were not articulated clearly by our women respondents in Dar es Sa-laam.[2] Evidently more important are views of health transformed not only in colonial times but especially after Independence by the socialist state with its emphasis on health development. A good example is the *Mtu ni Afya* (Man is Health) adult education campaign which was broadcasted over four months and covered a range of issues in community health.

As we argue in more detail elsewhere (see Obrist 2004a), women have learnt in school that hygiene forms part of the do-mestic skills *(maarifa ya nyumbani)* which every mother, wife and Christian woman in charge of a healthy home should learn (Fiedler 1983: 321). These ideas were reinforced under Nyerere as hygiene came to be considered as an integral part of *mambo ya maendeleo* (development issues) (Fiedler 1983: 12). Most probably already mothers of the women who participated in our study in Ilala Ilala, and certainly the women we talked to, had internal-ized health education messages linking cleanliness with health, and it seems plausible that these ideas have become embedded in broader discourses on domestic skills, Christian virtues, disci-pline, progress and modernity. These discourses have been, and continue to be, spread through various media and institutions, and have contributed to establish the responsibility for domestic health as an integral part of female gender identity.

Research is also a social experience shared by the investiga-tor and the respondent. Study participants consciously or uncon-sciously respond in ways that might be of interest to the researcher. Since we used the term *afya*, a concept which has become closely associated with medicine and public health, and were somehow connected with a health project *(mradi ya afya)*, we probably

---

2   Most probably, the Islamic tradition of Arabic medicine has been much weaker in Dar es Salaam (and, indeed, in most of Tanzania) than in Lamu, Mombasa and other old centers of the Swahili culture. As we described in a previous chapter, Dar es Salaam was founded towards the end of the Swahili commercial empires, and soon became a colonial city.

evoked certain, rather than all, possible responses about health in a more general sense. Moreover, we specifically asked about "health in the home" *(afya nyumbani)* since we were interested in local understandings of "household production of health" (Berman et al. 1994). Again, this focus elicited certain ideas about health, while neglecting others.

Still, the evidence presented in this chapter shows that women in this neighborhood of Dar es Salaam have access to and command of a body of basic knowledge derived from public health. They are aware of the common urban health risks including water-born diseases, inadequate nutrition and malaria transmission routes. They emphasize problems related to all three features of urban vulnerability mentioned by Moser (1998): Environmental hazards (pollution vs. cleanliness), commoditization (need for cash to pay for basic necessities and services) and social fragmentation (neglect vs. care). Women are further clearly able to recognize bodily and mental signs of good health and illness, although many found it difficult to discuss them in an abstract sense. It was easier for them to elaborate on what they do for health in the household.

If we apply the analytical approach suggested by Foucault (1984: 32–39), however, we recognize that this kind of knowledge, rooted in health development frameworks, is also a code of values and rules justified by biology and other sciences. As pointed out earlier, lay persons usually cannot reenact in their minds how these facts were established, even if they "know" what is "good" or "bad" for health. This is also true for women in Ilala Ilala who follow IEC messages.

Our argument is not about the inadequacy of women's health knowledge and activities measured against biomedical standards. Rather, we claim that individual women do not just command knowledge or behave according to fixed values, rules or positions that can be measured as determinants. They are reflective actors and moral subjects who position themselves vis-à-vis available frameworks of interpretation or codes of conduct. We have already mentioned that individual women formulate multifaceted ideas about health. No two women made the same statements. They drew on a spectrum of existing ideas, selected different elements, weighted the relationship between these elements differently and thus constructed their individual views. Still, all statements root in common understandings. Women only expressed divergent views when it came to body image and to "big" vs. "slim" as an embodiment of health.

Several women made critical statements about the applicability of public health ideas in their particular everyday reality. They questioned whether one should talk about "good health" in connection with people like themselves who lack basic requirements such as financial means and water. We argue that in this sense "medicalization" in Dar es Salaam has been only partial, or delayed, and puts people, and especially women, into a paradox situation. Women have learnt to see many aspects of their everyday life as linked to health, but at the same time, their living conditions constrain them when putting this knowledge into practice. This difficulty, for instance with regard to boiling water, has also been noted by the TzPPA (2002/03: 95). Women's response options seem less limited by the amount and range of health information they receive; on the contrary, they are often exposed to too much and contradictory health information. While health development discourses are kept alive, not least by development organizations, the Tanzanian state has not really been able to institutionalize and implement these discourses, for instance through the maintenance and extension of basic urban infrastructure or the provision of adequate and reliable services. These limiting factors, themselves consequences of the interlinked forces of environment, economy and governance, restrict women's response options.

Viewed against this background, women's varied use of public health knowledge begins to make more sense, and agency comes into sharper focus. Like other studies (Lock and Kaufert 1998a), we found that some women try hard to follow public

173

health messages, others comply only partially, and still others seem to be indifferent. The boundaries between these groups are not clear-cut in terms of education level or religious affiliation, and even within groups we find diverse stances. "Ambivalence coupled with pragmatism" (Lock and Kaufert 1998b: 2) seems to be a wide-spread position women take, also in Ilala Ilala. It reflects the extent to which women are prepared to commit themselves to a "healthy life" under the given circumstances. Additional aspects that come out from our empirical data are the powers of personal habit and social custom in shaping women's responses to health prescriptions transmitted through various institutions. We have further seen that women's notions of health are also a result of embodied experience, faith and trust in medical traditions.

Our discussion has shown that health in this particular urban context is not the polar opposite of "disease" but rather of "vulnerability to health risks". Women in Ilala Ilala are critical of a narrow medical view of health because their daily experience reminds them of their exposure not just to disease but also to the risk of going hungry, not having water in good quality and sufficient quantity and thus lacking a clean place to live in. At the same time, they represent themselves as actors, not victims, and describe in many different words and phrases how they "try hard" (*kujitahidi*) and "make sure" (*kuhakihisha*) to achieve at least minimal standards of nutrition, hygiene and care to ensure their own health and the health of their family. Whether they succeed in putting public health knowledge to socially acceptable and effective use on the individual and household level is to a large extent shaped by morality and pragmatics – as well as by financial means and social support, as the following chapters will further elaborate.

4   Health practice within the household

In the previous chapter we have seen that local understandings of everyday health practice in this lower middle-class neighborhood of Dar es Salaam are very much shaped by health development discourses. The emphasis is on body, mind and living conditions including basic needs, cleanliness and care.

This chapter examines how health practice is organized within households. We shall see that women's concerns center around problems which have already been recognized in predominantly feminist studies on urban survival strategies in Dar es Salaam (Koda 1995, Tripp 1997) and other cities (González de la Rocha 1994, Hoodfar 1997). Changes in the global economy and, more particularly, the urban crisis have affected gender relations within the household as women have become increasingly engaged in productive work to complement the inadequate incomes of their husbands. As many of these studies have argued, the consequences of these economic and social changes are complex and have repercussions on women's reproductive labor and responsibilities. In the perspective presented here, both productive labor and reproductive work are integral parts of health practice. The crucial question thus is how health practice has been affected by these changes in gender responsibilities. We do not just consider men and women as individuals but as members of households. We investigate how women respond to these changes and whether these responses are effective and socially acceptable.

We take the health activities as a lead which women in Ilala Ilala consider as relevant for domestic health *(afya nyumbani)*. These include the generation of income, food provision, personal and domestic hygiene, child care and health care. We use the concept of "task-centered interactions" to empirically investigate how people organize themselves in each of these activities. As the name of the concept implies (see Chapter 1.6), we consider health activities as tasks which have been culturally assigned to certain categories of people by virtue of gender, age, household membership or another principle of social organization. Moreover, we assume that persons who have been assigned responsibility for certain tasks interact with others in their performance.

Such an approach facilitates empirical investigation of gender norms in comparison with lived gender relations. It is a well-known fact that gender models rarely accurately reflect male-female relations as they are enacted in day-to-day life (Ortner and Whitehead 1981: 10). Rather than assuming health practice to be determined by fixed gender rules, we expect individual women's course of action to be a product of their own moral stances as well as of overt or covert negotiations with the husband and other household members.

Household health decision making has to be understood in the context of these interactions and negotiations. With Douglas (1992: 11, 40) we assume that people, and especially women rarely make decisions on their own, especially if costs are involved. They consult with the husband, children or relatives, take their advice into account and try to reach a consensus. Often, these negotiations are not verbal but enacted; women do certain things and respond to actions of others.

A focus on these interactions allows us to investigate cooperation and conflict within domestic units. As Sen (1990) has pointed out, the household can be seen as an arena of "cooperative conflict". While household members collaborate and face outside forces as a unit, harmonize their activities and thus act as a corporate group, they may, at the same time, have conflicts of interest regarding the allocation of resources or the division of responsibility. Since the overall approach of our study is resource-oriented, we shall pay particular attention to cooperation and support. What kind of support can women mobilize within the household to maintain or improve health and to reduce vulnerability?

In the household interviews we asked about the gendered responsibilities for the health activities women identified. We complement these data with observations and casual conversations in naturally occurring situations. For the presentation, we rely again on quotes from women's statements and from our field notes. We prefer this mode of presentation to a generalized narrative because it gives direct insights into the diversity and heterogeneity of women's points of view.

4.1 Negotiating responsibilities

Gender division of responsibilities

The division of responsibilities *(majukumu)* presented in Table 11 reflects the dominant gender model. The husband is responsible for generating income and for covering all the major health-related expenses, especially the costs incurred in the provision of food, water and health care. The wife is responsible for all the other health activities. Responsibilities of the husband towards the household are thus mainly defined in terms of productive work, while women's responsibilities refer to reproductive work.

In the cultural and social sciences, "reproductive work" has a variety of connotations. They range from the process of biological reproduction, that is child birth and lactation, to physical reproduction, namely the daily regeneration of the labor force through cooking, cleaning, childcare, looking after the old and sick and running a household, to social reproduction which refers to the raising of culturally and socially competent members of society (Moore 1988: 52, Brydon and Chant 1989: 10).

The subsequent sections examine, whether and how this socially defined code of values and rules is enacted in everyday life.

Table 11
Gendered responsibilities within households

Health activities	Wife	Husband
To generate income		X
To provide food		
To pay for food		X
To buy food	X	
To cook food	X	
To ensure cleanliness		
To pay for water		X
To fetch water	X	
To clean rooms	X	
To wash the dishes	X	
To do laundry	X	
To take care of children		
To provide body care	X	
To mind children	X	
To provide health care		
To pay for health care		X
To give and seek health care	X	

Generating income

In our discussion of the urban household economy in Ilala Ilala (see Chapter 2.4) we saw that almost 70 percent of the women pursue an income generating activity. Many women are petty traders (33 percent) or long-distance traders (5 percent), and quite few are wage earners (19 percent) and small scale entrepreneurs (12 percent). Our discussion further showed that the majority of these women still consider the household to depend on the husband as main breadwinner, as defined in the Swahili gender model (see Table 11). A smaller group claimed their household depended on both parents, and another small group insisted that the household depended on themselves. Not surprisingly, most of the women in the first group did not earn an income, while nearly all the women in the second and third group did.

The question now is how the relationship between productive and reproductive work influences women's daily routine with regard to health practice. To analyze this question, we first have to determine women's work patterns and then establish step by step how these patterns influence each health activity. To give an example, we shall ask how women who are not involved in income generation organize food provision compared to women working full-time away from home. And with whom do women in each group interact to have this task accomplished?

In this analysis, we do not distinguish between the four household types in our study sample. We shall rather see with whom women interact in whatever type of household; based on these data we then examine differentials in household types.

We begin our analysis by looking at the daily routine of women who are not involved in productive work (see Table 12). These women commonly get up around five or six o'clock, cook breakfast for their husband and children and make sure that the elder children get ready and leave for school. After breakfast, they clean their room and do the laundry, always keeping an eye on the smaller children who stay at home. Most of these tasks are performed in the communal courtyard. While they do their house work, women chat with other tenants of the same Swahili house. Once the clothes hang on the line to dry, women take a shower and dress up for the market. They spend about two hours walking to the market, chatting with people, buying the daily necessities and carrying them home. After a brief rest, they prepare lunch. When the elder children return from school, mothers serve lunch, eat and chat with the children and then take a rest on the verandah. Around four o'clock, the women iron the clothes, cook dinner and wait for the husband to come home. After dinner, the women get the children ready for bed, and around nine o'clock, the adults go to sleep.

Table 12
Women's involvement in productive work (N = 100)

Women's work patterns	%
Not involved in productive work	31
Works at home	30
Works part time away from home	14
Works full time away from home	25

An exception to this pattern is the daily routine of several, comparatively well-to-do women, often of Arab or Indian origin, who employ somebody to do the reproductive work. They get up early, do the prayers and then go back to bed. Around 8 or 9 a.m. they have a leisurely breakfast and then pass the time until lunch, for instance with phone calls to friends, planning social activities or overseeing the house helper. In the afternoon, they have a nap, rest and watch television or go out for a visit. They often prepare the main family dinner themselves, eat and chat with their husband and children, watch some more television and then go to bed.

At the other end of the spectrum are women who work full-time away from home. The following self-accounts illustrate the daily routine of a nurse, of a long-distance trader and of a school teacher who also runs a tailor shop.

Nurse:

I get up at 5 a.m., wash some clothes, prepare porridge for my youngest child and prepare those who go to school. At 6.20 a.m., I leave for the hospital and do not return until 3.30 p.m. After work, I do some laundry and rest while waiting for the evening meal. We eat at 7.30 p.m. and go to bed around 10 p.m.

Trader:

After waking up at 6 a.m., I have breakfast. Then I give instructions concerning the housework, lunch and dinner and leave for the market to sell the maize. I close my business at 6 p.m. By the time I return home, I am tired. I take a shower, eat dinner and go to bed.

Teacher:

At 5.30 a.m., I clean the house, wash myself and prepare tea for the children. At 6.45 a.m., I leave with my children for school. From 10 to 10.20 a.m., during the break, I rush home to give tea to the smaller children. Then I return to school until 2 p.m. After school, I go home and prepare lunch. From 3 to 4 p.m., I wash clothes and prepare a sauce that I will serve at dinner and again for lunch the next day. At 5 p.m., I go to the store to supervise the work of the tailors I employ. At 6 p.m., I close the store, go home and cook rice. While I prepare the food, I look after the children taking their shower. Around 8 p.m., I iron the next day's clothes. This is a must everyday. Then we eat and rest.

Although their daily routine differs in detail, all women in this group face a similar situation: They have little time for housework and childcare. Most of them leave home early and return late.

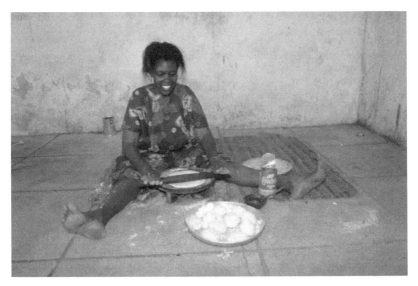

Plate 11
Many women earn some money by selling homemade food.
This woman prepares *chapati* (Photo: B. Obrist van Eeuwijk).

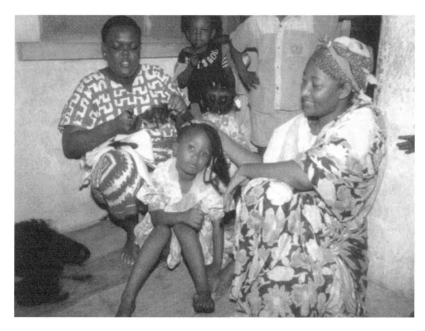

Plate 12
Women skilled in plaiting hair can earn a small income
(Photo: B. Obrist van Eeuwijk).

In between these two poles of the spectrum, women make various arrangements to squeeze some income generating activity into their daily routine of domestic tasks. One group of women uses the home for productive work. The following examples describe a day of a food vendor (see Plate 11), of a traditional healer and of a local hair-dresser (see Plate 12).

Food vendor:

I normally get up at 5 a.m. and start making the dough for the *chapati*. The charcoal stoves have to be ready by 6 a.m., otherwise my clients who are employed in town would go to work without breakfast. At around 10 a.m., I do the cleaning and then prepare lunch for my children. In the early afternoon, I prepare *kachori* and bring them to a nearby shop. Then I start cooking the evening meal, and the day is over.

Healer:

At 7 a.m., I prepare tea. Afterwards, I do the dishes, go to the market or buy the daily necessities in the nearby shops. My husband does not really like me to go out. While I continue with the house chores, I often have to stop in the middle because somebody needs my services as a healer, and I attend to my customers. Lunch is ready at noon, and we have dinner around 7 p.m.

Hair-dresser:

At 6 a.m., I get up, sweep inside and outside the house and wash the dishes and clothes. Then I prepare breakfast and eat with the children. Later I go to the market and prepare the sauce for the whole day. When a customer comes over, I plait her hair, but this is not always the case. In the evening, I cook *ugali*. Then I bath the children and bring them to bed. If there is a customer, I plait her hair, and it may well be midnight before I go to bed.

The accounts of these women vividly illustrate that women's productive and reproductive work is often closely interconnected (Moore 1988: 49). Their choice of income generating activities is often limited by their skills, the assets at their disposition and the reproductive responsibilities they have.

Another group of women works part time away from home. The following accounts describe the daily routine of an ice cream maker, a fish seller and a long distance millet trader.

Ice-cream maker:

I get up at 5 a.m., take the ice cream blocks out of the freezer and put them in special buckets. Then I prepare breakfast, clean the house and mix water and sugar for the ice cream I want to sell the next day. At 10 a.m., I carry the two buckets to Kasulu Primary School and start selling until 3.30 p.m. After coming home, I eat and finish the preparation of the new ice cream blocks. Then I check with my girls about dinner. This is my work schedule. I have hardly any time to rest.

Fish seller:

Everyday except for Sunday I have to go to the ferry market around 8 a.m. in the morning and return around 11 a.m. After that I do the cleaning and cook lunch. Then I fry the fish and take them out for selling. Towards the evening, I come back, wash the children and cook. I rest only after dinner.

Trader:

> I wake up around 6 a.m., wash the clothes and dishes. Then I prepare breakfast and eat with my children. Around 10 a.m., I go to the market for the day's relish, come home and cook lunch. In the afternoon, from about 2 p.m. onwards, I go to Tandale where my brothers-in-law help me to sell the millet.

Although two of these women have a home-based enterprise, they sell their products elsewhere. Their time for housework is limited to a few hours in the morning and in the evening.

These findings again illustrate the diversity, heterogeneity and flexibility of daily life in Ilala Ilala. It would be difficult to find even two women with exactly the same daily routine and work pattern. Still, these four work patterns capture differences in the daily routine which seem relevant for the organization of everyday health practice. With the exception of the relatively well-to-do women, we expect women who are not engaged in productive work to carry out most reproductive work themselves. Women who work some hours, half day or all day away from home will probably depend more on the practical support of others.

We can further assume that women without an independent income rely on the financial support of their husband and that they consider him not only as main breadwinner but also as head of the household. This raises the question, whether women's dependence on men decreases if they earn their own money. If this assumption is correct, women who work full time would either say their household depends on the parents or on herself.

However, only the first assumption is born out by evidence (see Table 13). Nearly all women without productive work say their household depends on the husband, although some of them made critical remarks. The only exception is a woman who has an independent income from renting out rooms. Women who work full time away from home, however, are distributed across all headship categories. In fact, the majority of the women who earn an income, whether they work at home, part time or full time away from home (44 out of 69, that is 64 percent), attribute

184

headship to the husband, even though some add a "but". Smaller groups of these working women speak of parental or female headship, respectively.

Table 13
Dependence and women's involvement in productive work

| Women's productive work | Household dependent on | | | |
	Husband	Husband but...	Parents	Mother
Does not work	24	6	–	1
Works at home	21	4	3	1
Works part time away from home	7	3	3	1
Works full time away from home	8	1	8	9
Total	60	14	14	12

These findings correspond with those of feminist researchers mentioned earlier (see Chapter 1.4). Women's income alone does not lead to fundamental changes in male-female power relations. In other words, the fact that a woman pursues an income generating activity, even if she is employed as secretary, nurse or bank clerk, does not necessarily make her an equal partner with her husband in terms of headship and dependence. Feminist researchers have suggested that other critical factors like women's self-perception of their status and personal power as well as political recognition of gender issues have to be taken into account (Bruce and Dwyer 1988: 8, Moser 1993: 27). In the next section, we shall see that some women in our study sample mention still another aspect.

Providing food

According to the traditional Swahili gender model, the husband is the breadwinner *(mtafutaji)* and the wife is the cook *(mpishi)* (see Table 11). The husband not only pays for food, he goes to the market to purchase it, and he picks up occasional food gifts along the way. When women speak about food provision, they differentiate between these aspects and explain who pays for, who buys and who cooks food.

Paying for food

If women do not engage in productive work, the husband gives a daily, weekly, by-weekly or monthly allowance, and the wife has to budget. In our sample, there are only two exceptions to this rule. One woman contributes money from income earned by renting rooms, the other woman just stopped working as long-distance trader and lives from her savings.

Women who work at home or work part time away from home commonly "help" their husband and spend the money they earn on food and/or fuel for cooking. The following example illustrates such a joint arrangement and shows how tight many of these household budgets are:

> He normally leaves me with 1000 Tsh or 700 Tsh per day. This is usually not enough. I may add up to 2000 Tsh a day. The good thing with my husband is that he always buys things for breakfast before he leaves. On the other hand, although we are guaranteed to have breakfast, sometimes he does not leave any money for lunch or dinner. I thus realized I had to find ways to generate extra income in order to back him up. It is not that he does not want to leave any money, no, sometimes he does not have it.

This woman actually adds twice the amount her husband gives her. Still, she does not complain because she knows that he is not unwilling but unable to provide more money for food purchases. Other women face a similar problem:

> My husband gives me money for food, but I also take from my business. We use 2000 Tsh per day. He sometimes leaves me with 3000 Tsh per month. Then I really have to budget.

> It's not as if he leaves 1000 or 500 Tsh every day. If he has, fine, if he has not, also fine. To add is important, if what he left is not enough.

> For the small things, I am responsible. He is responsible for the big things like finding the money for the children's education and future life. When I have not earned anything with my business, my husband gives me at least 500 Tsh a day.

Among the women who work full time away from home, some do not contribute to food expenses but pay for the education of their children or use the money for themselves.

> My husband pays for the food. The money from my shop pays for the education of my children.

> He leaves 4000 Tsh everyday. I don't add anything. With my own money, he says, I should solve my own problems.

Several other women "back up" their husbands like the women in the previous category, not all of them voluntarily.

> Of course, I am not staying at home so that he would give me money before leaving for work in the morning. When he gives me 5000 Tsh, he wants it to cover the whole week. I have to add because this amount is not enough.

Still others claim that parents should collaborate in sharing food expenses, and a few are the main breadwinner.

> In my house, there is nothing like the husband giving daily allowances. The salary that comes first goes to food and other needs.

Two points of more general interest come out of this discussion. First, studies on income generating often infer that women who engage in productive work automatically contribute to food expenses. Our study shows that this question has to be investigated, not assumed. We found four patterns: The husband covers food expenses; the husband pays, and the wife "helps"; the parents share the costs; or the woman provides the money.

The second point is that even women who actually contribute more to daily food expenses than their husband reject assuming responsibility (*jukumu*) as main breadwinner. They insist that they only "help" or "back up" their husband.

Every now and then, I help him, when his pocket is not okay; but he is responsible for food. […] Adding is necessary.

This is his responsibility. My responsibility is to cook. I do not pay for food. […] There is no standard measure. It is not guaranteed. However, when he gets money, he can leave 1000 or 1500 Tsh per day. Adding is necessary.

The husband is responsible for that, but when there is no food, I provide my own money because when you ask him, he will say, you are also working.

Such statements should not be interpreted as an expression of low esteem of women's status and personal power, as sometimes suggested in the literature (Bruce and Dwyer 1988). These women in Ilala Ilala refer to their right to depend on the husband, a privilege they seek to guard. In her research in a Muslim community of Cairo, Hoodfar made similar observations. She points out that "the most important privilege Muslim women have is the unquestioned right to economic support from their husbands, regardless of their own financial resources" (Hoodfar 1997: 270). In the rapidly changing urban context, women had a "vested interest in reminding their husbands of the 'words of God' that made them economically responsible for their families" (ibid). Many women in Ilala Ilala pursue the same interest.

In Cairo as well as Dar es Salaam, many women and men nowadays negotiate gender responsibilities concerning food expenses. Women's decisions and course of action have to be interpreted as a result of these overt or covert negotiations. If the husband does not provide enough money, the wife may decide to take up an income generating activity or, if she already has her own income, her husband may request her to take over some of the costs. Many women respond by occasionally contributing money but declaring it as help. Others negotiate to contribute to other household expenses, not to food. Still other women agree to share responsibility for food provision, and in a few cases, the husband earns enough to tell his wife to spend her money on her personal expenses.

Buying food

Women without a productive activity now often go to the market themselves. However, better-off couples tend to follow the traditional gender model. The wife either sends her house helper, or the husband takes care of shopping, especially if he owns a food store or works at the market. In four households, the husband still brings home all the food, in many others, he brings food gifts, for instance fish, fruit, bread, milk, meat or beans.

For women who spend some hours on an income generating activity, it is difficult to find time for buying food. They often ask their children to assist them. Younger children are not sent to the market, only to nearby stores. In several households, father and mother collaborate; he buys staples, especially if he owns a bicycle or even a car, and she does the daily shopping for relishes.

Another shift of responsibility occurs, if women work full time away from home. These women commonly employ a house helper or, if they have adolescent daughters, they rely more heavily on them, whether these are their own or foster children. Before they leave in the early morning, they instruct them what to buy, and leave the money needed for these purchases. Only in one case does another relative, namely a mother-in-law, provide support in daily shopping. She belongs to an extended household.

Which member of the family goes to buy the food depends, first of all, on the agreement between husband and wife. If the husband leaves this task to the wife, she can decide whether she goes herself or sends a child or a house helper. This decision is influenced by her work pattern, but also by the other members who live in her household. If she has only small children and no house help, she has no choice but to do it herself. Another important aspect she has to take into account is her budget. Women's decision margin is narrow, if husbands, for whatever reason, barely provide for daily necessities, and widens, if the husband is able and/or willing to provide generously. In our sample, about 13 percent of the women can make a comparatively free choice in buying food. The following statements illustrate the range of options in households of comparable size.

> The amount depends on how much he wakes up with, sometimes 500 Tsh, sometimes 1500 Tsh. So the task is with the mother. The amount is normally small. When you see, there is little money, you buy the cheapest relish for that day. [Nuclear household, three children]

> My husband gives money, and the house helpers go to the market. I only go myself, if I need something special. He leaves 3000 Tsh per day, but everything that is needed [the staples, cooking oil etc.] is available in the house. [Nuclear household, three children, two house helpers]

> My husband sends money, and if it is finished, I give him a telephone call [he lives in Kigoma]. He transfers lump sums of 300,000 to 400,000 Tsh for the children's school fees, electricity and other things like food, whenever I let him know. [Polygamous household, two children, two house helpers]

If the wife has an income generating activity, she may have some more leeway for decisions. On the other hand, as we have seen, husbands may give less money and insist on a contribution from the wife.

Cooking food

Women in Ilala Ilala very much identify with their responsibility as cook *(mpishi)*, whether they are involved in productive work or not. The common pattern is that women in charge of the household negotiate with other female members to take turns in the kitchen. Better-off housewives and women who work full time away from home leave breakfast and lunch to the house helper and prepare the main family meal (see Plate 13). In households with several daughters aged ten and older, a special day may be assigned to each of them, or one daughter may cook lunch, another dinner. Sometimes, a daughter prepares the staple, and the mother cooks the sauce (see Plate 14). Women regard the involvement of their daughters and foster children as education. Cooking is considered as a highly valued female skill, and mothers train and supervise their daughters in the preparation of

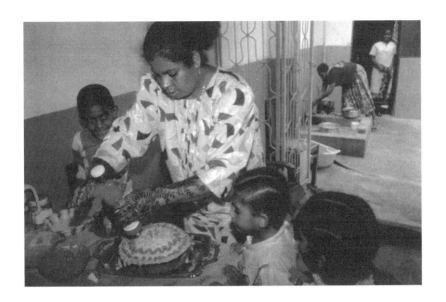

Plate 13
A comparatively well-to-do woman prepares a birthday cake. In the background,
a woman from a neighboring house fetches water from a tap (see Chapter 5.2,
Photo: B. Obrist van Eeuwijk).

different meals, if they find the time to do so. In a few of the
extended households in our sample, a mother-in-law occasionally helps with the cooking.

With regard to this as well as all the other health activities,
we always asked about the reason for assigning responsibility to
this gender and not the other. Although we did not expect highly
illuminating answers, we were curious to hear whether women
just accept the current model as "custom" or whether they critically reflect about it. We classified the answers in "practical reasons", "cultural values", "personal character or habit" and "gender critique" (see Box 2). When it comes to cooking, we found
that two men assist their wives, but the majority of women do
not even consider it as a possibility.

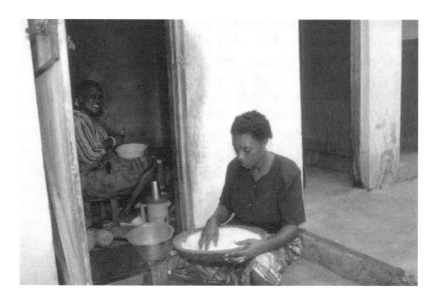

Plate 14
Mother and daughter share the task of cooking. On the right is the entrance to the toilet and the shower (Photo: B. Obrist van Eeuwijk).

In fact, even the pragmatic statements can be interpreted as refer-ring to cultural values, namely to a "legitimate excuse" (Finch and Mason 1993: 102). Because men's work is highly valued by the society, they are exempted from reproductive work. The same value is not necessarily attached to women's wage earning work. Many women carry out reproductive work before leaving for the office and after returning from work. Similarly, it is also a cultur-ally accepted value that people have different characters and hab-its, but apparently, this value is also gendered. If we invert the statements, they mean that men are not expected to do domestic work, and if they do so, it has to do with their character. The great majority of women in Ilala Ilala is not critical of this gender divi-sion of responsibility. They take it as the way things are, and a few refer to them as Swahili values.

Box 2

Women's rationalizations why men avoid reproductive work

Why men don't	Practical reasons	Cultural values	Personal character/habit	Gender critique
...cook	When he leaves in the morning, he does not come back until 10 p.m. When is he going to cook? He is not around most of the day, and the house helper was hired also for this job.	It is our custom (*desturi*) that a married man does not enter the kitchen. The wife is there to cook for him. In our culture, it is an insult (*matusi*) to let men cook. It is not a normal thing for a man to cook, once he is married.	It is not his character (*tabia*). He does not have this habit (*kawaida*).	Our men, when they get married, they think they have a servant. You know them! Our men still succumb to the old ideology (*kasumba ya zamani*).
...fetch water	He is also busy, not that he is lazy. He provides the money, and I buy it.	A man cannot go out and fetch water. It is better for me to do it. Getting water is my and my children's responsibility, not his.	He does not have that habit (*sifa*).	He would never do such a thing! When a man marries, he will depend on his wife for such services. He will tell you that's women's work.
...clean rooms	He is really busy looking for daily food (*posho*).	Letting your husband clean the house is not a Swahili characteristic (*tabia za kiswahili*). It is European, and it is very bad. This is the duty of the wife and mother. Maybe if she travels, he may do it. ... The mother is the keeper of the home (*mtunzaji wa nyumba*). The person who takes care of the home (*mlezi*) is the mother.	Things of cleaning? Don't tell him! If possible, he would like me to brush even his shoes.	When a man gets married, he knows that his wife will do all the housework.

193

Ensuring cleanliness

Fetching water

In water provision, the husband is responsible for covering the expenses, and the wife has to make sure that water in sufficient quality and quantity is available in the household. Women however increasingly "help" their husbands in addition to fulfilling their own responsibility. As two women put it in a focus group discussion:

> All that concerns water falls into the mother's domain *(yanamhusu mama)*. The husband is involved in giving money or paying the water bill. If I ask my husband for money to buy water, he gives it to me. On other days, I have to use my own money.

> When the husband leaves money for food, the woman makes the budget. If money is not available, we fetch water during the night from our neighbors. If there is enough money, we may buy from those boys who pass with water carts.

In another focus group discussion, a man made a similar statement:

> The husband pays. The one who earns money. If no water comes out of the pipe, you have to buy water. If the wife has an income generating activity, fine, we help each other.

Although women regard the husband as responsible for paying, they were less defensive in their statements about water than in those regarding food, probably because they blame the government and administration rather than the husbands for the problems they face in daily water provision. Since this neighborhood was reconstructed under the Slum Clearance Program, each house is connected to the main water system, but many taps run dry (see Chapter 2.3). Since women have to leave the household to get water, we shall examine these interactions in the next Chapter.

Here we focus on the social dynamics within the household. Most women have to economize not only in food but also in water provision. Even small amounts of money can make a difference, as the following notes from home visits illustrate (Appendix 2).

> Maria has a problem with water. If she buys from a street vendor, she has to pay 700 Tsh for a container. This is too much, so she tells her daughter to go and get water at Bungoni [the next neighborhood]. It takes her four rounds until the big steel drum used for water storage is full.

> Latifa sits on a stone collecting water from a main pipe they had dug up illegally. She says they had to dig deep because the pressure was very low. "You need a trick to get water from this pipe, that's why I come here myself. It takes a long time to fill the bucket, but I have to stay here because many people look for water today. We can either queue here or go to the next street. There you pay 10 Tsh."

Many women try to save small amounts of money by investing time and physical labor in fetching water, even if it is at night.

Again we find that women negotiate with their daughters and house helpers for assistance. If women are not engaged in productive work or work at home, they either fetch water themselves or send their own or foster children to do so. Even small children contribute their share, as we often observed. Women working part or full time away from home rely more on their daughters and house helpers. In three households, mothers have completely delegated this task to children.

> Monika's children often help her with the household chores, especially when it comes to water. Even the very young one can carry a small pail or a pot. They walk across the street, fill their pails and pots, come back to the house and pour the water into all the available containers, until they are full.

Although young boys assist in fetching water, this task is primarily assigned to daughters. The majority of the adolescent and grown up men are not involved in the actual carrying of water, at least not in public. If there is a tap in the house, they may lend a hand. Those few husbands who fetch water with the children do so because their wives have backaches. Illness is one of the few culturally accepted excuses for a woman to neglect her responsibilities.

Several husbands occasionally buy water from street vendors, for instance if their wife and daughters are tired and insist on their support. Women explain this division of responsibility mainly in practical terms (see Box 2).

Cleaning rooms

Cleaning is considered a female task. Except for the few better-off ladies, women without productive work or home workers sweep and mop the rooms themselves or ask their children and house helpers to do so. Women working part time away from home rely more on their daughters, those who work full time more on house helpers. As in the case of cooking, the mother, daughters and house helpers often share the work. Women who are involved in productive work may clean only on weekends. Others have set up a schedule, assigning certain days to their daughters and house helpers. Most women seem to accept or resign to the fact that cleaning is a female task (see Box 2).

Doing the dishes

In the household interviews, we did not systematically inquire into dishwashing, but most women have mentioned it when describing their daily routine, and we have frequently observed this activity (see Plate 15). Many women start the day by fetching water and then clean the rooms, wash the dishes and do the laundry. They either do it themselves or, if other women live in the household, they divide the tasks between them. Women who live in a well-to-do household or are busy with their income generating activities usually delegate this task to a daughter or a house helper.

Doing the laundry

Mothers who do not work or work at home often do the laundry themselves or receive assistance from their daughters. Two women assign this task to the house helper. The pattern again changes, if women spend more time away from home. They either share this task with their daughters or the house helper, some even leave it to the latter. A frequent arrangement is that the mother washes her own clothes, those of the small children and the father, and the older children do their own (see Plate 16). House helpers spend much time washing and ironing children's clothes (see Plate 17). If a relative lives in the same household, he or she is responsible for her own laundry.

Husbands often do some washing. Two men relieve their wives who have small babies and no one to help them with household chores. Others wash their own clothes, bring them to the dry cleaner or do their laundry on the weekend. In a few cases, men help women with their own and the children's clothes.

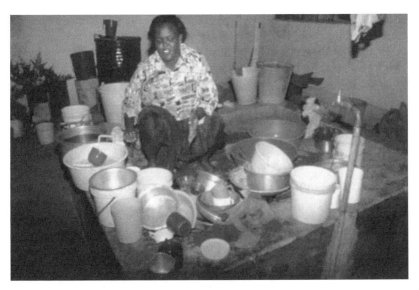

Plate 15
Washing the dishes in the *karo* can be a major task (Photo: B. Obrist van Eeuwijk).

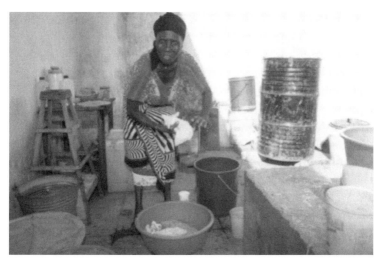

Plate 16
The grandmother does the laundry using many different containers and basins. She helps her granddaughter who is at work
(Photo: B. Obrist van Eeuwijk).

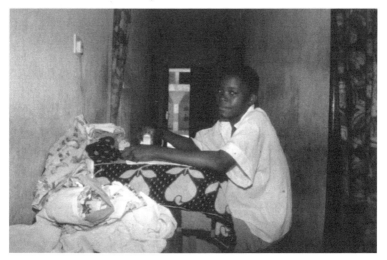

Plate 17
The house helper Zubeida irons clothes in the corridor
(Photo: B. Obrist van Eeuwijk).

198

Taking care of children

Providing body care

Babies and small children are bathed, groomed and dressed several times throughout the day. Mothers staying or working at home usually provide body care themselves, those working away from home do so early in the morning and again in the evening but during the day they have to leave this task to house helpers. In the morning most women supervise their elder children as they get ready for school. They keep an eye on them as they take a shower, clean their nails, groom their hair, brush their teeth and put on a clean and ironed school uniform. Adolescent daughters and house helpers often help the younger ones to brush and plait their hair and to iron their clothes.

Women who work and have nobody to assist them often find it difficult to take proper care of their babies and small children, even if they work in or near the home, as the examples of Pili and Lilian illustrate. Pili is a widow and runs a single-parent household with five children. Her eldest daughter is ten years old and does the cooking when she comes back from school.

> When we arrive at 11 o'clock, Pili is busy frying fish. She sits near the house, breastfeeds her two-year-old son and chats with a friend. When she gets up to check the fish, the boy starts crying. She tries to soothe him and then takes some water to wash him down, just next to where we are sitting. She wraps him into a *khanga* [a wrap around cloth worn by women], sits down, lifts him to her lap and tries to make him sleep. After a while, she carries him inside and puts him on the bed. Then she goes back to her business.

Lilian lives with her husband and a daughter in a family house. He works as a tailor in the city and assists his wife in her business of selling fish and fruit. The daughter goes to school and helps the mother with cooking. The other children live with relatives in others parts of Dar es Salaam.

Lilian has a little boy who is about one year old. He is always dirty when we visit. Although Lilian lives in a family house, nobody assists her in childcare. She herself is so busy with her work, she either does not notice or simply does not have time to take better care of the boy.

These examples stand in sharp contrast to that of women who have more time, support and money. They or their helper bath the children with soap, use baby powder, change their diapers, dress them in clean clothes and carefully plait their hair into different styles (see Plates 18–22).

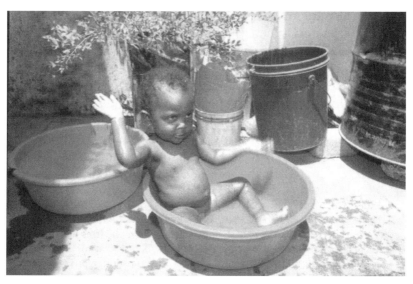

Plate 18
Baby Latifa enjoys her bath (Photo: B. Obrist van Eeuwijk).

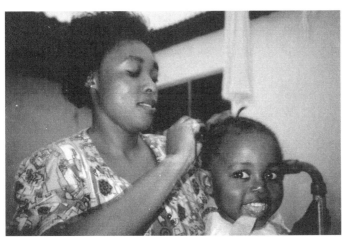

Plate 19
The mother carefully plaits the hair of her small daughter
(Photo: B. Obrist van Eeuwijk).

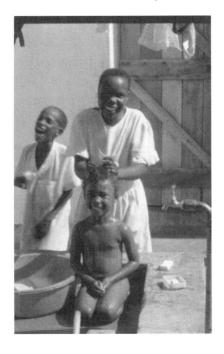

Plate 20
The house helper Amina
helps the smaller children
to take their shower
(Photo: B. Obrist van Eeuwijk).

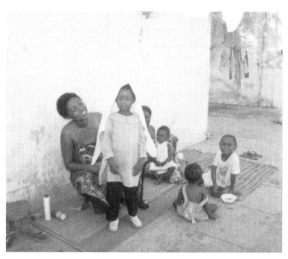

Plate 21
The mother minds the babies and prepares the elder daughter
for nursery school (Photo: B. Obrist van Eeuwijk)

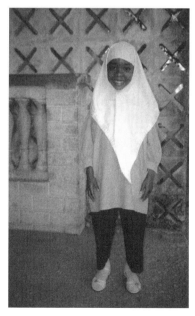

Plate 22
Amina looks smart in the new uniform
of the Moslem nursery school
(Photo: B. Obrist van Eeuwijk).

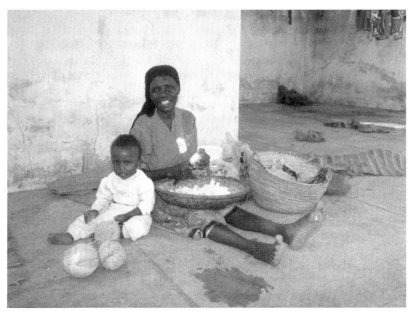

Plate 23
Grandmothers often have the task of minding small children (Photo: B. Obrist van Eeuwijk).

Minding children

Minding children is a task shared by all women living in a household. In two extended households, grandmothers are much involved in looking after toddlers (see Plate 23). Many women do not allow children to venture far. They keep them in the courtyard and forbid them to play on the street. One often hears them yelling: "Amina, where are you? Come here!" *(Amina uko wapi? Njoo hapa!)* They often complain that it is not safe for children to play outside because of open garbage holes, passing cars, broken glass and pools of dirty water. The following observations underline this point.

> Sada goes out of the room calling Omari, the young boy, and brings him in. He looks very dirty. Sada asks her daughter for the washing basin and

water and pulls out a soap dish from under a couch. Salim [her husband] says: "Omari needs a warm shower; he has a running nose." Sada does not agree because she is going to bath him indoors and will not let him outside again afterwards. She sighs and tells us: "Bringing up a child in our environment is very difficult. It is almost impossible to keep my child clean. Sometimes I just close my eyes. Pressing Omari to put on his shoes is a big struggle. Anyway, he wears them only for a short time and then he throws them away. Like the other time, when he was playing in the mud outside. I was not surprised to find him drinking dirty water with a dirty tin. It is nearly impossible to keep children from playing in mud and dirt. […] I used to get a headache when I had the twins. When one of them saw the other one heading to the toilet, he would follow. All I could do was shout every now and then because at that time, I had to prepare *chapati* and *sambusa* for a hotel at Kariakoo. […] The life of the children is in God's hands because no single mother can protect her child from all the dirty things in our environment […], perhaps only those who own a big house and an area for their children to play in a compound like that belonging to Mzee Makaranga [the construction contractor]."

Some women actually find it too hard to look after their children and pursue an income generating activity. If they have relatives who are willing to support them, they foster them out.

Nuru tells us that she does not keep time for either lunch or dinner because one of her small daughters lives with her sister and the other one with her mother in other parts of Dar es Salaam. "Because of my business, I cannot take care of small children."

Other women rely primarily on their older children to look after the small ones and take in foster children to help them.

The children are playing outside as we come to the house where Joyce lives. Victor, the child of the husband's brother, carries the baby of Joyce on his hip. We go up to him and ask for Joyce. He tells us that she is in town and will be back immediately. The baby does not look as smart as she usually does. She must have eaten something giving off color because her mouth and parts of her face are red. We enter the house and find dirty dishes lying on the floor. […] Joyce returns shortly afterwards and sees the dirty dishes. She gets angry with Victor and threatens not to give him any dinner. The boy replies that he had to spend much time carrying the baby because she did not fall asleep. He could not continue with the other activities. Joyce is not satisfied. She tells him that the baby is dirty and that this is the reason why she could not sleep. She orders him to put some water on the electric stove and fetches a washing basin. When the water is warm enough, she starts to bath the baby with soap, grooms her and dresses her in clean clothes.

As these observations show, it is not an ideal solution to leave child minding as well as other household chores to adolescent children. Yet, for many women this is the only option they have, if the husband's meager contribution to the household economy forces them to pursue an income generating activity.

Providing health care

In the household interview, we asked each mother, whether a member of the household had been sick recently *(siku za karibuni)*. More than two-thirds of the mothers (N=71) answered in the affirmative. In some households, more than one person had been sick, for instance two children or one of the parents and a child (see Table 14). Even if this is only a small sample, the figures indicate that people suffer a high burden of disease in Ilala Ilala.

Table 14
Number of sick persons[1] by social category

Social category	Number
Mother	8
Father	6
Children	65
Relative	
Grand-mother	4
Brother-in-law	1
Sister-in-law	1
Sister	1
Brother	1
Total	86

1 People who had been sick "recently", that is in the past few weeks before the interview.

The gender division of responsibilities in health care follows the general pattern of health activities which involve costs. The husband is responsible for paying, the wife for organizing and carrying out the task. There are, however, some variations from this pattern. Grown-ups take care of themselves if they are physically capable and/or have the financial means. If a child falls severely ill and has to be admitted, the husband is often involved in making arrangements and bringing the child to the hospital. The husband is also in charge if the patient is his relative, for instance his mother.

An interesting point is that relatives figure more prominently in this than in most other health activities. Firstly, they are mentioned as members of the household who have a health problem. Most of them live in extended households, but in a few cases, they have come for a visit in order to get treatment in the city. Secondly, relatives are mobilized if the members of the household cannot master a situation. The story of Fatuma exemplifies this point. At first, Fatuma took her sick child to the nearby hospital and went to neighbors for additional help. When the child's condition got worse and had to be admitted to hospital, the mother mobilized support from her husband as well as from her mother-in-law and her sister who live in other parts of Dar es Salaam.

> When we arrive at her house, Fatuma tells us, she is fine, except for the fact that her daughter Zawadi had fallen ill the day before. She has diarrhea. Fatuma and her children had taken her to Amana Hospital, but they could not get the prescribed medicine. So they went to the neighbors, and they gave them Septrine tablets. Salima gave the child half a tablet.

> At our next visit three weeks later, we meet Fatuma's mother-in-law who had come from Mtoni because Zawadi was ill again. She had to be admitted to Dar Group Hospital. Fatuma's husband works for the public transport company UDA, and this is the hospital where UDA employees and their family members get treated for a reduced rate. Her father had arranged for her to be admitted last Sunday. She has malaria. One of Fatuma's sisters is staying with her in the hospital to provide the services expected from relatives. Her mother-in-law came to support Fatuma with housework and child minding. Children of Fatuma's sister-in-law come to in-

quire about Zawadi's improvement, but they leave immediately after lunch. Fatuma says: "That's life. Instead of going to the hospital to see Zawadi and to find out whether they can help they just come here and pass by." After lunch, Fatuma prepares rice cooked with coconut milk for Zawadi. She then gets ready to bring the meal to the hospital.

Even though these nieces passed without offering their help, Fatuma was very lucky indeed to receive support from her relatives. In the next chapter, we shall have a closer look at the role of social networks in health practice; here we keep the focus on social dynamics within households.

Since we were particularly interested in decision-making dynamics in health care, we included two open-ended questions in our household interview: We asked women who made the final decision *(uamuzi wa mwisho)* about treatment seeking in the health episode they mentioned, and why it was this and not another person. Here we shall only discuss decision-making with regard to children under five years of age.

Table 15
Health care decisions in relation to women's work patterns

Women's work pattern	Wife decides	Parents discuss	Husband decides
Does not work	8	4	4
Works at home	11	3	2
Works part time away from home	3	2	1
Works full time away from home	2	1	1
Total	24	10	8

Our data show that several and partly inter-related decision-making patterns exist in Ilala Ilala (see Table 15). A first group of women (N = 24) reports that they themselves have the final say if a small child falls ill. Their explanations vary. Some argue they have to do so because their husband is not available during the day.

I am the one who takes the child to hospital. If my husband is not around, I have to use the money he left for food or any spare money I can find. I cannot wait until he returns from work. I take action.

If a child develops a fever during the night, the husband usually accompanies the wife to the clinic.

We felt that she had high temperature during the night, and she was listless. My husband and I went to the clinic to check for malaria parasites, and they actually found them.

Some women feel their husbands do not care enough; they have to take the initiative. Others consider themselves as the person who knows the condition of the child. The subsequent examples show that women can impose their decisions on their husbands, even if they earn only little money and say their husband is the head of household.

I am the one who knows the condition of my child, whether it is good or bad. I do not wait to be told. (Woman works at home, male headship)

My husband tends to ignore and gets angry quickly, for instance if the children do not take the prescribed medicine. He says, it is up to them. So I am the one who fights on with them, pushing them to take medication, when they are sick. Therefore, I do not even wait for his approval. I just buy the required medicine and give it to them. (Woman works part time away from home, male headship)

He sometimes says, there is no money. We should only buy drugs. But I am strong and take the child to the hospital first and then bring him the prescription. He can then search for the drug. I do not like buying drugs by guessing. (Woman works at home, male headship)

A second group of women (N = 10) discusses the illness with their husband. The boundary between the first and the second group is not rigid. Whether the mother takes action or discusses it with her husband often depends on the severity of the illness.

It depends on the severity of the illness. If it is very severe, then we have to discuss. If the child is ill and continues playing, then I do not have to consult him. (Woman works at home, male headship)

> We sort of cooperate when one of our children is sick. So sometimes, I decide and inform him later. At other times, I wait for his consent especially if the illness is serious but, at the same time, does not need immediate action. Then I wait until he comes home. (Woman works part time away from home, male headship, wife helps)

> There are some diseases, if they take more than three days, we sit down, discuss and advise each other. We do not quarrel. We understand each other. We look at the weight of the illness. (Woman works part time away from home, male headship, wife helps)

As these examples show, joint decision-making for these women does not only mean to voice their opinion but also to receive advice. In this and many other contexts women emphasize advice as an important form of support.

In the third and smallest group (N = 6), the husband is the decision-maker *(mwamuzi)*. The conditions of these children were no worse than those of the others. Most women in this group had consistently strong views about the husband's authority as head of the household.

> He is the head of this house. I cannot decide for him, I have to listen. (Woman works at home, male headship)

> The mother cannot have the last say by herself. The father is responsible for what should be done with his child. (Woman works full time away from home, parents share headship)

> I participate in giving advice, but he decides, if we should do this or that. (Woman does not work, male headship)

What is surprising is that most women reporting an illness of a small child present themselves as main decision-makers. A smaller number seems to share this responsibility with their husbands, especially in severe cases, and only a few women describe their husbands as decision-maker. These examples indicate that women's statements about dependence and headship in the household are a poor indicator for decision-making power in childhood illnesses.

A question we did not address in the interview was what happens if a small child develops a sudden fever and the parents

– or the mother in single-parent households – are away at work. According to our observations, it is beyond the capacity of most adolescent siblings and house helpers to take action on their own. Some mothers leave precise instructions, for instance to ask an adult person in the same house or the neighborhood. In some cases, the children just wait for the mother to come home.

Also for women who run a small business, the sudden illness of a child causes many problems. This happened, for instance, to Nuru.

> Nuru greets us saying that we are lucky to find her because she just got back from Amana Hospital. She had been there since the previous night. Nuru and her husband took the child for treatment, and the doctor suggested the mother and child should stay on for the second injection. The child had very high temperature and was vomiting. They had not realized that she was sick until late in the evening.
>
> Nuru asks her son to bring the tablets [Chloroquine and Aspirin]. When he brings them, she puts them in the mouth of her sick child. The child vomits, and the mother exclaims: "Oh no, where are we going to get another dose, she has vomited everything. We have not yet bought the [Chloroquine] syrup that was prescribed because I did not go to my business. And now she will not get any medication until I have earned some money."

Nuru's husband is a retired clerk whose pension is only a small contribution to the household economy. Since Nuru could not pursue her income generating activity while she stayed with the child at the hospital she now has no money for medication. If she continues to take care of the sick child, she will not be able to earn any money. The only option she has is to ask her husband and children to take care of the child while she goes back to her work.

Women like Nuru and their families were particularly hard-hit by the decision of the national government and city administration to introduce cost sharing in health care. As we argued earlier (see Chapter 2.1), it is not the individual reforms but their cumulative effect and the general urban economy that take a heavy toll on people with low incomes. These people are not only exposed to more health risks and, consequently, ill more often than people living in more favorable environments, they also carry a heavier practical and intellectual burden in mastering illness episodes.

4.2 Receiving and giving support

In the discussion of gendered interactions, we have repeatedly referred to ways in which women negotiate assistance in reproductive work with other female members of the household, mainly with their daughters and house helpers. In order to learn about women's own views on this subject, we asked them a set of open-ended questions in the household interview: "Who among those you live with supports you to maintain health in the household? How do they help? And why does their help assist you in improving the health of the household?" *(Nani unaoishi nao ambao wanakusaidia ili afya ya familia iwe nzuri? Msaada gani? Kwa nini msaada huu unakusaidia kuboresha afya nzuri nyumbani?)*

Table 16
Support in health practice within the household (multiple answers)

Health activity	Husband	Children	House helper	Other relatives
To generate income	21	4	–	1
To provide food	22	7	9	4
To ensure cleanliness	21	50	8	–
To take care of children	11	10	10	7
To provide health care	13	1	–	–
Total	88	72	27	12

To our surprise women regard husbands as main providers of support in all health activities except for those related to cleanliness (see Table 16). They provide many examples of close interaction with their husbands. Concerning income generation, women point out that the financial support from their husbands allows them to get basic necessities for health maintenance and care.

> He tries his best to search for money, so that we can get food and other care. He pays for our clothes, medical drugs and the medicine for washing the mosquito nets [insecticide for treating bed nets].

> He makes sure there is food and provides for other daily needs of the household. We are able to get food and things like soap needed for cleanliness.

Husbands bring food gifts and thus relieve their wife in shopping and budgeting.

> He sometimes brings the relish for the following day, and this enables me to use my time for other things.

> When he has money, he buys a tin of flour, and this reduces the "sharpness" *(makali)* of budgeting. He may also bring two or three coconuts.

Men further provide practical support, directions and advice in tasks related to cleanliness and child care.

> In the evening, he sometimes baths the children, or when he sees their clothes are dirty, he tells them to take them off and helps with the washing.

> My husband helps with small activities, for instance carrying the baby when I am busy cooking.

> He helps in alerting the children to things that are not good for their health, for instance not to eat dirt or other things that are dangerous to health. He gives directions.

> When he finds the place dirty, he shouts: "Why this?" Or he says we should not drink water that is not boiled. Or when he sees a child has bathed and plays with dirt, he spanks her. He insists on things.

While the last statement portrays the husband as exerting authority, other women speak of their husbands more as partners.

> My husband listens to me, when I have a problem, and that is help in itself. He has now gone to the *shamba* [fields] in rural Dar es Salaam and will bring food from there.

212

> I get help from my husband like washing clothes, ironing them. If I have to work late in the office, he goes to the market. Then I only have to cook, when I come home.

> My husband is truly a great help. When I travel, he looks after the children, so that they eat, get washed and are clothed by the time I come back and find the house in good order and without problems.

Only four partnered women in our household sample complain that he hardly supports them.

> What my husband does, when I get ill is to inform the neighbors, so that they can come and prepare porridge for me and food for the children, nothing more than that.

> Reasonable help that comes from those I live with? I can say there is no such help.

> Nobody helps me. As you have seen, I do everything myself.

> In this household, nobody helps me. I wanted to register my child at school, but I could not afford it. There was no help whatsoever from this household.

These findings clearly show: If women talk about support, whether it concerns support they give to their husband or support they receive or expect from their husbands, they do not just think of financial matters. They portray themselves as helping their husbands to fulfill their responsibility for generating income, and they represent their husbands as assisting them in fulfilling their responsibility for domestic work. Whether this support is balanced out is another question and depends largely on the moral stance of individual women and men, that is on the way in which they interpret their conjugal relationship and roles.

More generally, this discussion of interaction and support reveals the multifaceted practical and moral dimensions of gender relations in health practice, and whether women interpret them in authoritarian or egalitarian terms. The spectrum of these interpretations is wide. Some women describe their husbands as representing the main authority yet providing support in daily domestic tasks, either through their own contribution or by hiring a house helper. Other women portray their husbands as partners, and still others say the husband insists on women's equal status but hardly supports them and their children.

It is self-evident that women living in a single-parent household cannot rely on a husband. Where do they get support from? Two women are members of compound households and receive help from the other tenants in the Swahili house.

> My fellow tenants help me very much because the way we live, we are like relatives. For example when I am sick, one tenant brings me to the hourly injections at Amana Hospital, and when I leave, the others take care of my child.

> We are all women in this house. We help each other like close relatives because none has a husband.

It is typical that these women mention examples referring to health care and childcare. In these two domains, women often enlist support from relatives living in other households. When it comes to the other activities, however, members of the household do the work.

Children provide much support to their mothers, especially in cleaning (see Table 16). They sweep, fetch water, wash dishes and clothes. Such assistance gives women time to attend to others things, primarily to income generation. Some women assign different tasks to their daughters and sons.

> My son fetches water, takes the small ones to hospital, when they are sick, and scolds them, when they go wrong. My daughter washes the dishes, sweeps and even cooks. She can also take her young brothers to the hospital, when they fall ill.

A few women mention that they send their children to the nearby stores or even to the market, and that they help with cooking and child minding. Two children help with income generating activities, and adolescent and adult children contribute to household income.

> The children, who live here, are involved in their small business. They buy their own clothes. For me it is only food now.

> The boys who live here, when they get their money from their activities, they give me 1000 Tsh each. For me that is great help.

Adolescent girls and boys employed as house helper are equally involved in cooking, cleaning and childcare.

> She cooks, cleans, serves the children food, eats with them, when I am away and spends time with them. She also looks after the house in my absence. She washes the dishes and makes the beds.

When we asked women specifically about support only few of them mentioned a house helper; they are clearly underrepresented in this table. Most probably, this can be explained by the fact our respondents draw a distinction between "help" *(msaada)*, which is considered as voluntary, responsibility *(jukumu)*, which is seen as a social obligation, and work *(kazi)* paid in cash or kind. House helpers are either fulfilling a kinship obligation or they are paid in cash or kind.

The relatives women mentioned as providing support belong to the extended or compound households in our sample. Those who help with childcare and cooking are mothers, mothers-in-law or sisters-in-law of the woman respondent. The exception is a brother. When he finds one of the small children wandering away from the house, he brings it back and gives it a spanking. A daughter-in-law helps with the cleaning, and a brother-in-law helps with money when the husband is away on business.

Our emphasis on support draws attention to the household as a corporate unit. Mother, father, children, house helpers and, in extended households, relatives collaborate in the daily struggle for health. This does not mean that the household is a harmonious unit without internal divisions, conflict or hierarchies, but it shows that all the household members are to various degrees involved in mastering the many problems they face.

4.3 Discussion and conclusions

This chapter focused on the role of the household in everyday health practice. The Household Production of Health framework suggested that the household is both a locale and a normative social institution in which resources can be mobilized to strengthen positive dimensions of health (Berman et al. 1994). The question thus is how social dynamics within the household shape women's response options to urban health risks. First we examined whether the reassessment and renegotiation of gender relations in the wider society also affect the social organization of health practice. How do women respond to these changes and are their responses effective and socially acceptable? Secondly, we investigated what support women can mobilize within the household to maintain health and to reduce vulnerability.

In our detailed analysis, we took those health activities as a lead which women themselves had identified as relevant for domestic health *(afya nyumbani):* generation of income, food provision, personal and domestic hygiene, child care and health care (see Chapter 3.3). For each of these activities we examined task-centered interactions.

Our findings confirm that changes in the economy which forced women to increase their involvement in productive work have an effect on the organization of health practice across household types. We see this as resulting from the close interconnection of productive and reproductive work in women's daily routine.

Not surprisingly, women who do not work or work at home perform most health activities themselves. If they have daughters of suitable age, they ask them for help in most household chores and gradually train them in tasks the society associates with womanhood. The few well-to-do women in these two categories assign most household chores to their house helpers. The pattern changes if women work part time or full time away from home. Especially in activities relating to cleanliness and childcare, the former rely increasingly on their children, the latter on house helpers.

Referring to Chant's (1991) work in Mexico City, we can thus say that the economic decline affects the household organization of health practice mainly in two ways. Women who contribute to household income either bear the double burden of productive and reproductive work or delegate at least part of the domestic work to children living in the same household, whether these are their own children, foster children or children employed as house helpers. A few women, we have seen, resort to the third option described by Chant, namely to foster out some of their children because they cannot care for them.

Studies in other cities present a similar picture (Moser 1998: 12). Women often assume a disproportionate share of the burden of adjusting to adverse economic circumstances. As we have documented for Dar es Salaam, they increasingly take on paid work in addition to their reproductive work, but men do not respond by taking on significantly more household tasks. Intra-household time management data confirm that men and women contribute nearly the same number of hours in productive work, women further spend up to 16 hours a week in reproductive work, excluding childcare because its workload is difficult to measure, while men average five or fewer hours a week. Women, in other words, spend consistently more time working than men.

The delegation of domestic tasks to one's own and foster children as well as house helpers deserves particular attention in a study on health practice. Previous researchers working in Dar es Salaam (Fidelis 1994, Campbell et al. 1995) have emphasized the vulnerable position of children recruited for domestic work. Furthermore, these children rarely have the experience and competence of adult women in terms of health knowledge and practice. This makes not only themselves but also the other household members more vulnerable.

If we focus on agency, it becomes clear that the division of labor and responsibility in everyday health practice reflects not just changes in the economy but in values and rules of the wider society which shape the interaction of women, men and children as members of families and households. The dominant gender model in our study sample is hierarchical and defines male identity largely in terms of household provision and leadership which are regarded as the main attributes of headship (see Chapter 2.4). Female identity is primarily constituted by women's activities as homemakers. Even though the majority of the women engages, in addition to their responsibilities as homemakers, in productive work and contributes often substantially to household income, the gender model of male headship persists.

Nevertheless, responsibilities for income generation and for covering costs incurred in daily health practice (see Table 11) have become a subject of negotiation between husband and wife. In some households, this may lead to conflicts, but most women in our sample present themselves as using "non-confrontational, non-threatening methods" (Obbo 1981: 102) in these negotiations. Indeed, the situation we found in Dar es Salaam in the mid-1990s resembles that reported by Obbo from Kampala, Uganda, in the late 1970s.

> Urban women, in order to gain wealth, power and status, not only worked hard but capitalized on the traditional virtues of submission and service and their roles as wives and mothers. In other words, women were changing their situation by means of non-confrontational, non-threatening methods (Obbo 1981: 102).

Many women in our sample insist that they only "help" their husbands to fulfill their responsibility for household provision and thus implicitly reject to assume this responsibility themselves. Especially Swahili women, i.e. women of coastal origin and/or of Islamic faith capitalize on the virtue of the mother as dependent homemaker and, as Hoodfar (1997: 270) has put it referring to women in Cairo, their privilege and unquestioned right to economic support from their husband, regardless of their own financial resources. Although, or perhaps just because some of these Swahili women in our sample are aware of the gender inequality sanctioned by the wider society, they try to make the best out of their situation by insisting on their right as married women. Women of other ethnic background and Christian faith also insisted on this right, and one of them referred to the Bible to justify her claim.

The notion of non-confrontational methods helps us understand why not only women living up to the traditional role as homemaker but also the majority of the women pursuing productive work at home, part time away from home or full time away from home (64 percent) attribute headship and thus the main responsibility for the household to the husband.

Smaller groups of working-women interpret their situation differently. The first group emphasizes the importance of helping one another in these times of economic hardship; they associate this with shared responsibility of the parents to provide and lead the household (see Chapter 2.4). Most women in this group are Christians from northern Tanzania. A second group of women has to take full responsibility for productive and reproductive work because they head single-parent households.

Women's positions toward gender models influence the ways in which they interpret their responsibilities, but only with regard to the health activities of income generation and of paying for food, water and health care expenses. Our data show that their responsibility for all the other health activities remains unquestioned. Hardly any woman considers the option of transferring some of these responsibilities to the husband.

Their positions may also be influenced by their very realistic fear of the high economic risk of separation and divorce. Moreover, marital conflicts and even domestic violence may have been underreported in our study in Dar es Salaam. Several studies in other cities have shown that domestic violence was prevalent, probably due to adverse economic conditions putting additional pressure on couples (Moser 1998: 13). What we have noted is that the increased reliance on children's contribution to productive and reproductive work has sometimes led to conflicts between parents and children.

While economic and social constraints create tensions and even inequity within families and households, the gender and intergenerational relations of household members are also "critical safety nets long before outside help is provided" (Moser 1998: 11). The women in our study very much stress the importance of support from their husbands, not only in financial but also in practical and moral dimensions. They consider this as "help" in the same way as they regard their own productive activities as "help" for the husband.

Adult relatives living in extended household were only occasionally mentioned, for instance a mother-in-law who helped with cooking or with childcare. This indicates that many health activities are carried out by the nucleus of a family based household, that is mother, father and children. In single-parent households the nucleus is of course reduced to mother and children. Those who can afford it extend this basic unit with a paid house helper.

Most women know from their own experience and/or observe among friends, neighbors and relatives how harsh life becomes in the city if the husband is either not able or not willing to provide support. This is exacerbated if women have only small children to support them in domestic work. If they do not pursue an income generating activity, their main constraint is money. If they are involved in productive work, their main constraint is time and energy. In both cases, they cannot provide proper care in a broad sense including food provision, cleaning, childcare and care for the sick.

In conclusion we argue that family values constituting the household as corporate unit are an often underestimated but highly relevant resource in everyday health practice. Women's interpretation of reciprocity and support may differ according to their specific situation and moral stance. What counts is that they can mobilize key values engaging all household members in a joint effort to take care of personal and domestic health. As the negative scenarios show, the most crucial elements in this joint effort are a husband who provides adequately, one's own engagement in an income generating activity and adolescent or adult household members providing support in reproductive work.

5 Health practice at the interface of household, social groups, networks and institutions

After examining the social organization of health practice within the urban household, we now look beyond this unit at the interface of the private and the public sphere. In the pursuit of their health activities, women obviously do not just interact with other household members but also with neighbors, relatives, and friends as well as with providers of formal and informal services. By tracing these interactions we aim to identify principles of social dynamics linking the household with broader groups, networks and institutions. The critical question is how social dynamics at this interface shape women's response options.

Many studies in Dar es Salaam (Mwami 1991, Tungaraza 1993, Lugalla 1995, Tripp 1997) and in other cities of developing countries (González de la Rocha 1994, Hansen 1997, Hoodfar 1997) have emphasized the embeddedness of households in wider social networks. They found that individual members of a household create social relationships for different fields and purposes. These networks provide a range of resources: contacts and information, help in terms of services, goods and money, loans, access to facilities, pooling resources for ceremonies or emergencies, moral support, training and apprenticeship and saving. Nowadays, they are often interpreted as safety nets or informal insurance networks and received much attention in research on poverty reduction (Moser 1998, Morduch 1999). While these studies offer many insights into diverse aspects of people's social and economic life in the city, they provide little information on the social organization of everyday health practice.

Of particular interest to our resource-oriented perspective is the question of support. Researchers working in Dar es Salaam previously referred to the pioneering work of Lomnitz (1977) in Mexico City. Taking up her concept of an "ideology of assistance", they argued that this ideology reinforces exchange relationships, particularly those between members of social networks (Mwami 1991, Lugalla 1995). What kinds of support do people give and receive in everyday health practice? And how does this support and assistance contribute to reducing their vulnerability?

Our approach encourages a new look at the relevance of social networks for health, redirecting attention from a normative discussion to lived practice. Rather than investigating people's formulation of cultural norms we have to gain a deeper understanding of rules that govern their everyday life. Moreover, in an urban context marked by dynamics and diversity, we cannot assume people to strictly adhere to rules but rather expect them to be involved in multiple overt and covert negotiations within their personal networks.

Again, we take up health activities identified by the women in our study and to reconsider them in terms of task-centered interactions. The key questions are: Which member of the household is considered responsible for particular tasks in health practice? Does this person interact with members of other households, social groups, networks or service providers in the performance of these tasks, and with whom and in what respects? And what types of interactions do people themselves conceptualize as support?

This chapter relies less on household interviews than on observations and casual conversations in daily life. To complement these methods and to gain deeper insight into matters of particular concern for this urban community, we organized several focus group discussions about the social organization of water provision and the collection of solid and fluid waste. Especially in these realms of daily health practice, the recent reforms we outlined earlier (see Chapter 2.1) have had a direct impact. To capture these changes, the focus groups discussions were repeated with the same social groups five years after the main ethnographic field research.

5.1 Organizing health activities

Generating income

The majority of our study participants are, to various degrees, involved in generating income. We now focus on women who are engaged in informal sector activities, sometimes in addition to formal jobs (62 percent), and investigate with whom they interact to perform these activities. What is striking is that most of these women present themselves as single actors receiving occasional help from their husband or children. They prepare food, make embroideries, mats or dresses, plait hair or work as traditional healer.

Only a small group (27 percent) explicitly mentions persons beyond the household with whom they interact in their small business. Most women in this group receive financial or practical support from relatives. Two brothers provided starting capital to set up a tailor's shop and to buy a freezer for making ice cream. An uncle constructed a shelter for frying fish. Other women collaborate with relatives in rural areas. Three women visit their home villages at the harvest of rice, maize or millet and sell the produce in Dar es Salaam. Another woman works with her mother on a *shamba* (field) at the outskirts of the city. Still other women share a business with relatives. They pool resources and labor, rent a room and a sewing machine and make clothes, run a small restaurant selling *pilau, ugali* and other local foods, or sell agricultural produce at the market.

A few women collaborate with people who are not kin. They have, for instance, an agreement with a shopkeeper. Some women bring their homemade food to be sold in a shop. Others get *khanga* (wrap around cloths) from a shop and sell them as retail street vendors. Still other women employ men to run their business, for instance young men to push water carts or to make dresses on a sewing machine.

We conclude that women in Ilala Ilala also create networks with relatives and non-kin to mobilize resources for income generation in the informal sector. However, if we compare these findings with those of Tripp (1994: 154–155) in an earlier study in Dar es Salaam, the percentage of women reporting such support in our sample is much smaller. In Tripp's study, 60 percent of the women received support outside the household, in our sample only 27 percent. This difference may be due to intra-urban differentials, but it is also possible that women underreported such support in our study.

What we have to keep in mind is that women engage in various other interactions as they try to solve their daily problems in productive work. They face many contingencies in the urban environment and often seek advice from relatives, neighbors and work-mates. How much money should they allocate to flour for baking buns in order to make a profit? What kind of fish should they get if the one they usually buy at the ferry market is sold out? What should they do if there is a power cut, and they cannot prepare ice cream for their small business?

Women's activities are also influenced by interactions in a much broader sense, for example by interventions of the government, as the following story illustrates.

> I had a stall for selling cooked food. It was demolished by people of the City Council. This was very sad because it was the activity which enabled us to pay for our daughter's school. Actually, it was not my own stall. It was owned by a rich lady who is my fellow tenant, and she asked me if I needed a place to do business. I accepted. I used to give her a certain amount of money as rent. But this business is no longer there now. At the moment I am cooking for the employees of a dispensary near my house, and sometimes I cook for some carpenters working close to my house.

As part of the economic and political reforms mentioned earlier, the city government destroyed the food stalls of street vendors who did not own a license (Chapter 2.1). This and other acts of repression during field research in the mid-1990s caused not only much emotional harm; they also made people lose faith in the government. Under such conditions, people have to organize themselves. In this case it was a better-off fellow tenant who rented the stall to this lady; after it was demolished, she started a home-based food stall serving meals to people working nearby.

The more general point we wish to make here is that even if many women in our sample describe themselves as single actors, they act in a web of social relationships which have influence on what they think, feel and do. It is in this sense that anthropologists prefer to think of individual persons as social actors, and this perspective also guides us in our emphasis on task-centered interactions.

Providing food

One of the key responsibilities with which women identify is being the main cook *(mpishi)* of the family. Most women interact with many other persons in activities related to food provision. Since the provision with food in good quantity and quality is a major concern and daily worry (see Chapter 3), we focus our discussion on specific relations women create in order to save a few shillings in food purchases.

During one of our visits, for instance, Latifa came with a shopping list for her house helper. She told her to go to a certain shop in Bungoni Street. When the girl had left, she explained to us that this shopkeeper allows her to buy staples like maize, flour and rice on credit, and she continued:

> The shop is also cheaper. The girl can get half a liter of kerosene for 100 Tsh. In other shops, the same amount would cost 120 Tsh. You know, 20 Tsh is a lot, when you have little cash. As long as I had my trade with Mombasa, I did not face these problems. Now I see cooking oil from Kenya or washing powder, and I cannot afford it. Life is difficult because money is a problem. Instead of buying a whole tin of cooking oil, I have to buy in small quantities from nearby shops, and the shop keepers want to make a profit.

Until recently, Latifa regularly traveled to Mombasa to sell second-hand clothes and made a good living, but she stopped her travels after meeting a new partner. Like most other women, she now has a tight food budget. As she says, "20 Tsh are a lot of money, when you have little cash".[1] If she can make a special arrangement with a shop keeper, it makes a difference in terms of the quantity and quality of food she can cook for her family. Other women have a special relationship with street vendors with whom they bargain for a good price. Some of these food vendors know the women by name.

> A street vendor comes over and calls out to each woman by her name. He carries a large wooden container full of tomatoes, onions, limes, carrots, green vegetables, pepper, small dried fish and fresh fish. The women come outside, greet him and start negotiating. Rose asks for *dagaa* [small dried fish], one heap of tomatoes and two onions. He sells the items for 300 Tsh with a discount of 50 Tsh.

Other women do their shopping in Kariakoo or other market areas where they know people who sell food at a low price.

We shall later see that women also receive occasional food gifts from relatives living in rural areas but, in general, our data confirm that food is a scarce commodity, even for these lower middle-class women in Ilala Ilala. During our follow-up visit five years later women still complained that food was a problem. Many new supermarkets have opened in Dar es Salaam selling food at prices these women cannot afford. A broad range of food is available in local shops and markets as well, yet only a small segment of the community has a comparatively free choice in terms of financial means to buy from it.

---

1   As these examples show, women's calculations deal with very small amounts of money; still, these small sums make a difference if the average budget for food, water and fuel is around 2000 Tsh (4 US$) a day.

Ensuring cleanliness

Fetching water

The daily water provision is the responsibility but also constant worry of women. At the root of the problem is the unreliable water supply system of Dar es Salaam (see Chapter 2.1). Since the demand for water exceeds the capacity of the urban water authority, and because much water is lost due to leaking pipes, water has to be allocated according to a rationing schedule. Every part of the city has its turn. Industries need much water during the day; private households are therefore mainly served at night.

Seen from within the neighborhood Ilala Ilala, supply of water seems even less regular. All houses built by the National Housing Corporation during the Slum Clearance Program were connected to the main water system in the 1960s and had communal taps installed in their courtyard. What is confusing is that some streets do not get any water, whereas others have a fairly continuous supply of it throughout the day and the night. People from "dry" streets go to "wet" streets to fetch water. Residents of Dodoma Street and Lindi Street, for instance, carry their pails to Chunya Street (see Map 4). But even in a "wet" street, not all the houses have water, as the following statements from women living in Chunya Street illustrate.

> We get water from the neighboring houses (Chunya Street 10).
>
> We fetch water in the third house (Chunya Street 12).
>
> We have a tap in the courtyard, and we can get water day and night (Chunya Street 15a).
>
> We have a tap but no water. We go to the third house at the corner (Chunya Street 15b).
>
> The tap in our house gives water (Chunya Street 19).
>
> We have an inside pipe, and it gives water (Chunya Street 21).
>
> We buy water from the second house. At the end of the month, we pay 400 Tsh (Chunya Street 25).

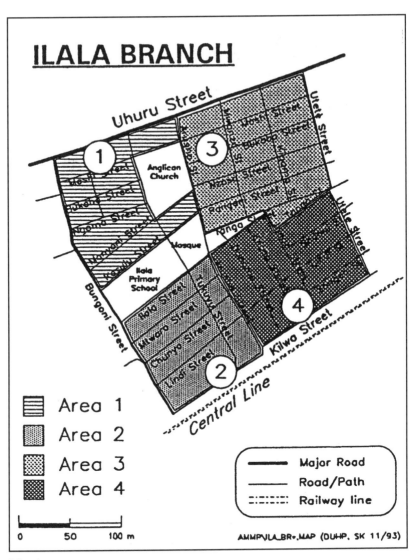

Map 4
Street map of Ilala Ilala

The residents of Ilala Ilala explain this uneven distribution of water by the fact that not all the houses are connected to the same water pipes. Moreover, water pressure in the pipes is low. If somebody installs an electric pump, he can draw water from the pipe system but then his neighbors have even less chance of getting water from their taps.

Whatever the reasons, the irregular water supply remained a mystery to us, even more so since the situation changed ever so often. At the time of our household interviews, houses with a steady supply were scattered over the whole neighborhood, and only a few of them had a pump. In our follow-up of twenty households, the situation often changed from one week to the other. The house where we were staying had no water for six months. Then, all of a sudden, the water started to run regularly for about two hours at midnight, though only from the lowest tap in the toilet. The water flowed very slowly; it took a long time to fill all the available containers for the next twenty-four hours.

All in all, in the mid-1990s women in Ilala Ilala had three possibilities of getting access to water (see Table 17): They either had to fetch water outside the house, they were able to draw it from a tap in the communal courtyard, or they could buy it from street vendors. Most women combined these options.

The majority of the women had to fetch water outside their house (see Plate 24). Some of them bought it from a neighbor or in a house located in another street. House owners or tenants who owned a water pump often charged a fee to recover their expenses. This fee ranged from 200 to 400 Tsh per month, or around 10 Tsh per container. This was cheap compared to the price of water sellers.

At least half of the women in our sample got their water free. They fetched it from a neighbor, in another street, the mosque or, if they had transport, from a friend or relative in another part of town. In front of a nice, new house, for instance, adolescent girls lined up every day in a long queue, each girl carrying at least one pail. The owner of the house had installed a long water sling that reached out to the street. He gave away his water free of charge.

Table 17
Options for getting access to water (multiple answers)

Options	Number of Households (N = 100)
Fetch water outside of the house	61
Fetch water from tap in the communal courtyard	34
Buy water from street vendors	29
Total	124

Such arrangements express a sense of solidarity among people who are usually not related but help one another in difficult circumstances. What is important, though, is that this "help" is not just there but subject to constant negotiations. Those who offer help often expect some favor in return or they may decide to help only occasionally.

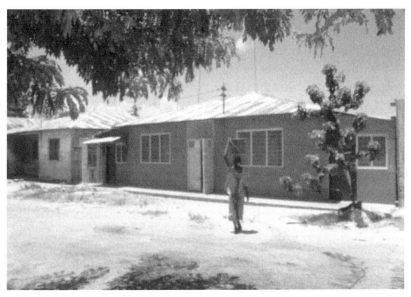

Plate 24
The majority of women have to fetch water outside of their house
(Photo: B. Obrist van Eeuwijk).

230

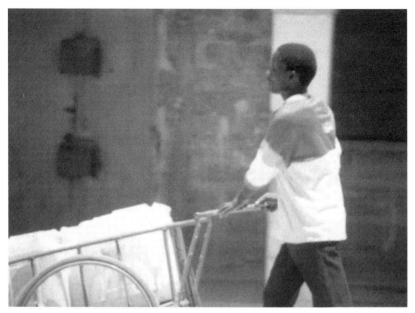

Plate 25
Those women who can afford it buy water from street vendors
(Photo: B. Obrist van Eeuwijk).

About a third of the women reported having a tap that gives water but, as mentioned above, a regular supply is not guaranteed.

> We have a tap that often gives water. When there is no water, we buy it from street vendors.

> Normally our tap gives water but now it does not. We have to fetch water at the school tap.

> Our water tap normally gives water at night. Fetching water is everybody's responsibility. There is usually a queue. Whoever wakes up in the household goes and lines up. If there is no water, we go to fetch it on the third street.

Women who could afford it bought water from street vendors (see Plate 25). The prices of street vendors fluctuated. If they had to go far to fill their water containers, the price doubled from 70 Tsh to 150 Tsh per container. A well-to-do woman bought eighteen

231

containers a day. She thus spent 1260 to 2700 Tsh a day only on water. This was more than the daily food budget of most households. Most women were forced to replace money by physical labor and to carry buckets of water, doing it either themselves or delegating this task to their daughters or house helpers.

Some women interacted with these informal service providers on a regular basis and established a social relationship that allowed them to buy on credit or at a discount. More often, however, the women and water vendors were strangers to one another and haggled about the price, as the observation during a visit to the home of Anna illustrates.

> A street seller passes with his small cart carrying only four water containers. Anna calls him and asks: "For how much do you sell your water?" The young man mentions 400 Tsh. Anna replies indignantly: "Only if it is Merry Water" [commercially sold filtered water]. The man explains: "I mean 400 Tsh for all containers." Anna is not willing to pay that much: "Then you better bring your water to the rich people who can afford it."

> Another street seller comes by just after the first one has left and says: "I want to give you this water". Anna jokes: "For free or do you want money?" He answers: "I am going to give it for a take-away price. How many containers do you take?" Before Anna can reply, the young man lifts the four containers from his cart and brings them to the verandah saying: "Just give me 280 Tsh because I haven't had my breakfast." Anna says: "You know your business well." She has money tied into one corner of her *khanga*. She gives 500 Tsh, and when she gets back her change, she tells us: "You see, we are going to get five *chapati* for breakfast out of this money."

Since Anna could not reach an agreement with the first vendor, she did not buy from him. The skilful bargaining of the second vendor made her decide to purchase his water. The good price she got then allowed Anna to buy some food for breakfast.

In principle, all tenants of a Swahili house contribute (*kuchangia*) to pay the bill of the urban water authority. In practice, only few households do so because their tap runs dry or gives water irregularly, not even according to the official rationing schedule. Some better-off women complain that even if they pay the bills regularly and directly talk to the clerks, they cannot rely on tap water. They might get it once a month and then on a few consecutive days. Most residents in Ilala Ilala see no reason why they should pay the bills. They do not get a service from the formal sector and have to spend money on services from the informal sector, although markedly smaller amounts. At the same time, the planned privatization of the city's water system scares them. What if there is a steady supply of water but at prices they cannot afford?

This situation has hardly changed by 2002. People in Ilala Ilala still complain that they receive bills from the urban water authorities now called DAWASA but not the service. Most taps do not give water unless an electric pump is installed, or the water comes irregularly and at inconvenient times. Owners of pumps still sell water to others. Those who can afford it still buy drinking water from street vendors.

What has changed is the provision of water for domestic use. After severe supply problems with water from Ruvu River, the Dar es Salaam municipalities began to draw groundwater. In Ilala Ilala, the government drilled four wells and equipped them with electric pumps for public use. Those who get their water from these public wells contribute to the electricity and maintenance costs by paying a regular price. At the mosques, well water is available free of charge. Several private persons have also bored wells which they operate with electric or with hand pumps. Some let neighbors use their well water for free, others charge a fee. Since people now very much rely on electric pumps, either to draw water from the pipes or from underground, they face serious problems if there are power cuts. In general, however, most residents of Ilala Ilala appreciate that they now have water in sufficient quantity for domestic use.

Drinking water remains a problem. First of all, water from the wells has a salty taste which many people do not like. Moreover, this water is not safe, especially if it is drawn from shallow wells. This aspect of water quality was a main concern and worry debated in all our focus group discussions and casual conversations. People are well aware of the fact that groundwater may be polluted because of leaking pit latrines and indiscriminate waste disposal. Now and again, there is an outbreak of water-borne diseases like cholera and dysentery. Most people agreed that wells do help but what they really want is good quality tap water in sufficient quantity as they used to have in earlier decades and as some people still have in more affluent parts of Dar es Salaam.

Cleaning the environment

Nearly all our study participants dwell in a Swahili house and share a common responsibility, namely to ensure cleanliness of the "environment" (see Chapter 3.3). "Environment" *(mazingira)* in this context means the verandah, corridor, courtyard and the communal facilities, namely the kitchen, toilet and shower.

This health activity is organized within the Swahili house community. All women who are in charge of a household form part of a rotational system called *zamu*. This social institution seems to have been invented by the former state party based on the well-known principle of reciprocity. The house owner is responsible for setting up a roster. If he or she fails to do so, the tenants organize themselves. A common pattern is for each woman to clean the environment for three days *(siku tatu tatu)*. If there are only two women in a house, they often take weekly turns.

When it is her turn, each woman is responsible for buying the water as well as the broom and detergent needed for cleaning. Male tenants who are single have, of course, no woman to represent them in the *zamu*. They are obliged to buy a broom or detergents or to pay the ladies for their services.

> The women of the house are responsible for cleaning the environment. The wives represent the husbands. Single men have to buy brooms for the cleaning.

In this house, I am responsible because most tenants are single. They have to pay for the brooms.

We, the women, do it in turns. Men go to work in the morning. Those who do not have a wife either pay the ladies for doing it for them or they buy brooms or detergents.

An often-heard rule in this context is:

Wives sweep the environment, husbands dig the garbage hole.

Only eight percent of our study participants said their Swahili house community did not follow the *zamu*.

Anybody in this house who is interested will clean the environment. We have no roster. A woman with children does it more often because she does not want to see her children enter a dirty toilet or eat where there are plenty of flies.

We used to have turns, but now people are spoilt. If you see the environment is dirty you clean it. Most of the tenants in this house are young men. They are hooligans. We are only two women.

The one who was in charge of the roster has died. He was a relative of the house owner. Right now, we don't have an arrangement. The one who is around does the cleaning.

Everybody in Ilala Ilala, and people of many other neighborhoods, know the rules of *zamu*, even if they do not follow them.

The interesting point here is that the Swahili house community, at least in principle, forms a corporate group for certain health activities. Each household is supposed to equally contribute to matters which concern the house community. Women thus not only interact with others as members of social networks but also as members of social groups. This is a new aspect of the urban social organization in Dar es Salaam which our focus on task-centered interactions has revealed.

Disposing of garbage

In the mid-1990s, many residents of Ilala Ilala complained that the City Council trucks no longer came to their neighborhood to collect garbage. They remembered the "good old days" of the 1960s and 1970s, when they kept their household waste in big drums, and City Council trucks regularly passed by to collect it. These services stopped in the 1980s.

The local representatives of the CCM party and the ten-cell leaders advised people to dig garbage pits around their houses (see Plate 7) and the *Bwana Afya* ("Mister Health", i.e. health officer) of the Ilala Ward passed by from time to time to inspect, whether the holes were properly covered. According to the official rule, husbands were responsible for digging pits, wives for disposing of garbage. In daily practice, however, most husbands contributed money and wives organized somebody to dig a hole or to collect the garbage. A few women did so on their own, even if they lived in a Swahili house; but the rule was that each Swahili house community acted as a corporate group.

The principles of social organization were similar to those mentioned above. Each household contributed in labor or cash. Often the tenants took turns *(kwa kupokezana)* digging the holes themselves. Sons or single male tenants occasionally volunteered. Sometimes they preferred to contribute money *(kuchangia)*, about 100 Tsh per household, and hired a casual laborer to dig the hole. Either the house owner, his/her representative or a particularly initiative woman became active, collected money from the others, went out to find laborers and negotiated the terms, or several women took turns in making the necessary arrangements.

The casual laborers women hired were often men who walked the streets and asked for work. Women paid them 300 to 1000 Tsh, depending on their negotiation skills. Some diggers received less money but were allowed to keep the sand and sell it. Others preferred to receive food for work. One of the big problems however was that the ground around the houses was already full with garbage that had not yet decomposed. There was no space left for new garbage pits. Every time they dug a new hole, they found garbage.

An alternative to digging holes was the utilization of collection services in the informal sector. Some especially poor men from Buguruni specialized in this service (see Plate 27). They walked the streets with a push-cart *(mkokoteni)*, collected the garbage from the houses and charged a fee ranging from 100 to 400 Tsh. It was not clear where they dumped the garbage; it was a rather secretive business because the City Council had banned the private collection of garbage by *mkokoteni*.

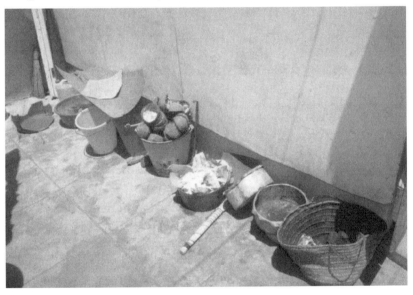

Plate 26
Women separate household waste in old containers. Coconut husks can be used as fuel, green waste will be thrown into garbage holes or given to collectors (Photo: B. Obrist van Eeuwijk).

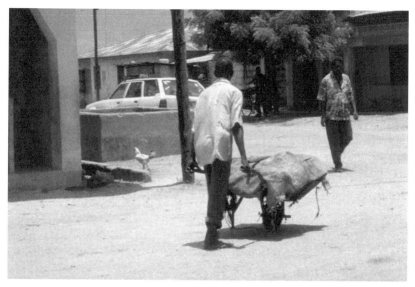

Plate 27

An old man collects garbage with an old cart. He covers the waste with an old rag because his business is officially banned (Photo: B. Obrist van Eeuwijk).

Many residents of Ilala Ilala did not abide to this regulation, mainly because the City Council failed to provide proper services. Their trucks occasionally drove through the streets of the neighborhood but they had very selective collection methods.

> The City Council truck stops in front of the restaurant and collects garbage. People from the neighboring houses quickly bring bags and pails and throw their waste into the truck. Soon the vehicle moves on and stops again in front of the house belonging to the construction contractor. His servants carry the garbage to the truck. After a few minutes, the car drives off and leaves the neighborhood.

This was not an exception but common practice. The restaurant owner and the construction contractor paid the drivers of the garbage truck for a whole month to come and collect from their houses. For a while, the truck drivers followed their order because they could earn good money. After they had failed to come

238

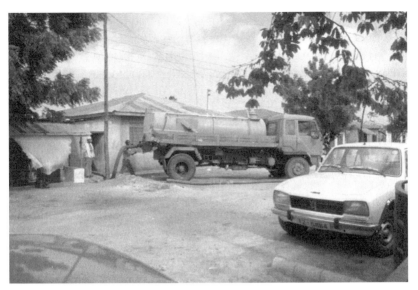

Plate 28
The City Council cesspit trucks serve only the better-off or better-connected households in Ilala Ilala. A long hose is laid from the truck through the entrance of the house to the cesspit tank to suck out the human waste (Photo: B. Obrist van Eeuwijk).

for a certain period, the construction contractor and owner of fourteen houses in Ilala Ilala set up his own garbage collection service by sending one of his cars to all his houses. The payment for this service was included in the rent.

The CCM party also organized a communal activity. On the open space in front of the party office, there was a big heap of garbage. All the men from the houses facing the open square were called to a meeting. It was agreed that each of them contributed to the digging of a large pit, where all the garbage could be dumped.

Yet not all people act on a principle of solidarity. Especially under the cover of the night, some people carried bags full of garbage and dumped it either into the pits owned by other people or in public places.

Five years later, people are no longer allowed to dig garbage pits. The municipalities have contracted private companies to collect garbage from house to house. In Ilala Ilala they have a timetable for most streets, and the trucks pass by twice a week. For this service the company operating in this area charges 2000 Tsh per month for each Swahili house. At the end of the month, company employees walk from house to house to collect the money. This is not an easy task because many people complain about the price, but if they refuse to pay, they can be taken to court.

Some focus group participants still remembered the 1960s when garbage was collected three times a week. Also, there was much debate about where and in what containers the garbage should be stored. In the old days, the government not only provided the collection services for free, it also distributed garbage containers with a lid. Nowadays, people can buy waste bins for 6000 Tsh. All agreed that this price was much too high for a box to keep garbage in, especially since containers of good quality are often stolen. Some people leave their garbage outside in polyethylene bags; others consider this unhygienic as these bags are easily torn apart, for instance by dogs, chickens or birds, and the contents dispersed.

Although they are still illegal, many people use the services of the cart collectors (*mikokoteni).* They are available at all times and do the job for little money. Today, the companies tolerate these cart collectors and allow them to use their local dumping site for a small fee. A few trucks of private individuals also collect garbage, but they tend to be even more expensive than the officially contracted company. All in all, most participants in our focus group discussions agreed that the new collection system was much better than the garbage pits.

Emptying cesspits

During the Slum Clearance Program, each house in Ilala Ilala was equipped with a cesspit tank and city trucks passed by regularly to empty them. As with garbage collection, the services had deteriorated to a point where City Council trucks served houses only selectively (see Plate 28). Five years later the situation was still the same. Without personal connections and bribes, it was impossible to obtain these services. Moreover, many residents complained about bad services.

> Last year before the elections, we called the City Council car. They asked for extra money for the fuel. It took three weeks for the car to come. Throughout this time, we had to knock on our neighbors' doors to use their toilets. When the car finally came, the hosepipe burst in the middle of the clearing process, and human waste was splashed all over. The tenants had to clean the house and the environment. The service men promised to fix the pipe and to return the next day in order to finish the job. They never showed up again.

People in Ilala Ilala have many similar stories to tell. What they report most frequently is that this method only cleans out the fluid waste and does not take out the solid waste in the lower part of the pit.

To organize the emptying of the cesspit tank is commonly considered the house owner's responsibility. He or she looks for people who have the necessary skills and pays them. Several women, however, report that their house owner does not care, for instance Christina and Joyce.

> After finishing her laundry, Christina asks us to come along and see where she drains the dirty water. She shows us the toilet. It is not roofed. She says all the rainwater as well as the wastewater from all tenants goes into that pit. The owner of the house does not care because he lives in Magomeni [another neighborhood of Dar es Salaam]. When the toilet is full, the tenants have to organize themselves.

> The previous year, Joyce tells us, the toilet was full to the brim. The situation was pathetic because the tenants had to go to their neighbors' houses to relieve themselves. When the owner of the house came for the rent, they informed him, and he promised to take care of the problem. But he did not return for a whole week. Her husband and other tenants decided to take action, because their families were suffering.

241

In most Swahili houses, the proprietor, his or her representative or – if they neglect their responsibility – the tenants themselves collect money from each household and then organize the services. Even in a family house with compound households, each unit is asked to contribute, either individually or taking turns (*zamu zamu*).

Most people in Ilala Ilala prefer to use informal cesspit services. They hire men who walk the streets and offer services called *kutapisha*, "to make the old toilet vomit", or *upakuaji vyoo*. The price for this service is a matter of bargaining. In 2002 it cost anywhere from 20,000 to 80,000 Tsh. In addition, the client has to provide cement and whatever building material is required. The workers dig a deep hole close to the toilet. Then they break the top of the existing toilet cesspit and make an opening wide enough for buckets to pass in and out. They fill these buckets with human waste and pour it into the new hole, until the cesspit tank is empty. It commonly takes them a whole day to dig the new hole, and another day to empty the cesspit. Before completing the work, they bring clean sand from the bottom of the old cesspit and show it to the client. Then they pour kerosene into the pit to kill the bad smell and reconstruct the old toilet using cement. The new hole is either completely covered or left partly open to be used as a garbage hole.

This activity is shrouded in secrecy, partly because it is officially banned, partly because the workers themselves do not like to be observed. The following observation underlines this point.

> When we come to the house of Victoria, two old men are busy digging a hole in the backyard. All the children eagerly observe what is happening. The husband of the other tenant brings a five-liter-container of kerosene and gives it to the old men.
>
> One of the men asks the girls and women to remove the stoves and what else they need that day from the backyard because they want to start working. The men leave the house and come back with a ladder and two buckets. A long rope is tied to the buckets. They call the husband and tell him to bring the keys to the door leading into the backyard. They order every-

body to leave and lock the door. According to Victoria, nobody is allowed to watch them. Some people say, these men work naked, others say they perform rituals to perform spirits living in dirty places like toilets before doing their job.

All the people we talked to agree that men using this local method are more reliable and do a better job than the City Council cars. They call them local experts *(wataalam wa kienyeji)*.

To empty cesspits is, of course, not a daily activity. In some houses, it has to be done every year, in others every two, five or eight years. The length of the interval depends on whether people use the toilet also as a shower. If this is the case, the cesspit quickly fills not just with waste but also with water.

In this activity, married women act mainly behind the scenes, especially if they are tenants. They complain to their husbands, to other tenants and to the house owners and thus indirectly exert power. Some women obtain information and contacts through their networks and even make first arrangements, with local experts knocking on the door to offer their services. Yet, it is commonly a man who takes charge, provides the money, organizes the required building material and supervises the work. If the house owner is a lady, she may well be the main actor, and single women make financial contributions just like husbands do.

Taking care of children

Childcare is clearly assigned to the female domain. As the previous chapter has shown, many women take in foster children or house helpers to support them in this task. Particularly women pursuing an income generating activity away from home are in need of such support. They leave their small children in the care of older children, foster children or house helpers or, if they live in an extended household, with a grandmother or another adult person.

Still another solution is to send children to live with relatives in the same neighborhood, other parts of town or even in another town. Four women in our household sample mentioned fostering out, two of them have already been quoted in Chapter 4. Their children live with relatives in other parts of Dar es Salaam because their parents cannot provide for them. During the cohort study, we learnt of two other cases.

> My father is my "big helper", nobody else, especially if my family has health problems, but also in other matters. My first born, for instance, is handicapped. He would not have seen a school because he cannot walk. My father bought him a wheel chair. They boy is now staying with him, and my father gives him everything he needs.

> What I consider great help is that my brothers take care of my children. Four of my children live with them in Tanga. They feed them, dress them and pay their school fees.

A few women have daycare arrangements with relatives living in the same house, the same neighborhood or in other parts of town.

> My mother-in-law helps me a lot in terms of cooking and caring for my children, while I am at work. She lives in the next house.

> My sister-in-law who lives in Tanga Street is my great help. Every morning, I bring my children to stay with her when I go to work, and on the way home, I pass there to pick them up.

If women go to the market or to town, they often leave their small children in the care of their fellow tenants or, if they live in a compound household, with their relatives.

> We live together with my brother-in-law and his wife. She helps me a lot. When I go away, I leave my children with her, and when I come back, I find them well and fed.

> When I go to the market or to town, I leave my children with my fellow tenants. They take good care of them.

Another woman pays the children of her fellow tenants to help her with child minding and domestic chores, while she attends to customers.

When many customers come to have their hair plaited, I ask the children in this house to watch my children and to do some housework. I pay them some small sum, like 500 Tsh.

A few women recount how relatives have taken care of them after childbirth. According to Swahili custom, a woman spends forty days "inside", that is in seclusion, and during this period, relatives are expected to relieve her from her normal duties.

All in all, it is difficult to judge to what extent relatives outside the household provide support in day-to-day childcare. On one hand, it is common practice to look after children of the same house while the mother goes for an errand or to provide support after childbirth; many women do not even consider it worth mentioning. This practice is based on a reciprocal exchange relationship. On the other hand, regular arrangements of daycare or prolonged care due to business activities seem to be the exception rather than the rule. Women who have a relative able and willing to do so emphasize that these people are their great helpers (see also Chapter 5.2).

A few women consider such support as a family obligation *(wajibu kwa familia)*, not as help *(msaada)* which is voluntary (see Chapter 4.2). Other women explicitly use the word *msaada*. This indicates that not only gender relations but also kin relations are reassessed and redefined in this rapidly changing urban context.

Providing health care

As mentioned earlier, relatives figure quite prominently in health care. Minor childhood illnesses are managed within the household but more severe cases involving children and especially adults often require interactions that are more complex. We already presented the case of a child suffering from acute malaria who had to be admitted to hospital (Chapter 4.2). Her mother mobilized support from her husband as well as from her mother-in-law and her sister, both of whom live in other parts of Dar es Salaam.

Not only in acute, also in chronic illness relatives play a part. In the previous section, we mentioned a grandfather taking care of a handicapped grandson. Another example is a grandmother from Temeke, a neighborhood rather far from Ilala, who took a chronically ill grandson to live with her. We learnt about this case during visits in the home of Sakinah.

> Sakinah tells us her son suffers from sickle cell disease and has to attend a clinic at Muhimbili Hospital every three months. She tells us, her first son had the same disease and was admitted to Amana Hospital, where he died. The grandmother has now intervened and taken the second boy to Temeke, where she feeds him with honey and sugarcane.
>
> When they came to Dar es Salaam, they lived a simple life. Her husband worked as taxi driver, Sakinah earned a small income with her *chapati*. She was even able to save some money. When her second son was admitted and diagnosed as suffering from this disease, she used up all her savings. They brought him to private hospitals and to traditional healers, but he is still weak and his skin is yellowish. Now her money is used up and they have decided that the grandmother should take care of him.

The example of this boy shows how prolonged illness depletes people's resources and makes them resort not only to different health care professionals but also to relatives and home remedies.

Another woman, Zuhura, told us of her niece whose illness was complicated not only for medical but also for social reasons.

> One day, Mwajuma visited and asked whether she could move in with us. She is the daughter of my husband's brother who lives in Nairobi. I accepted and later informed my husband. He agreed to take her in. Now, in fact, I did not know that Mwajuma was sick. She did not tell me, so I just assumed she had a quarrel with her friend in Oysterbay, where she was staying.
>
> Mwajuma planned to go and visit her father in Nairobi and needed a passport for that. My husband accompanied her to follow up on the passport. It was then that he noticed her bad cough. He asked her whether she had consulted a doctor, and she denied. He became concerned and decided to postpone her journey.

Mwajuma did not want to go for treatment. When my husband realized this and saw that she became unreasonably stubborn, he called a meeting of close relatives living in Dar es Salaam, namely her grandmother and two of her uncles. In this meeting, Mwajuma accepted to see a doctor but did not admit she had already done so. Only after the meeting, she confided in me and told me she had been diagnosed as suffering from TB.

My husband got very angry but nevertheless followed up her case and finally had her admitted at Muhimbili Hospital. She stayed there for two weeks until she was discharged. We were told how to separate her and the things she used in the house. Now she is fine and will soon visit her father.

Zuhura's husband called a meeting to discuss the case with relatives and to get their consent for the further course of action. By doing so, he not only asked them for advice but also to share the responsibility with him. This is an example of moral support, one of the resources provided by social networks mentioned in the literature.

A similar process occurs if adult relatives of the husband fall ill, for instance his mother. The husband's relatives get together and discuss what to do. As one of our study participants put it, it is the husband's responsibility *(wajibu)* to take care of his relatives; she is only an advisor and carries out what the husband and his relatives decide. If somebody on her side falls ill, her relatives get together to find a solution, and she is more involved than her husband.

Relatives also play a major role if a woman in charge of a household falls ill, as the case of Saada illustrates.

When we arrive at Saada's house, a middle-aged woman is there taking care of the household. We ask about Saada and learn that she is in Amana Hospital. She was suffering from acute malaria and had to be admitted. As we continue to talk, the woman introduces herself as Saada's sister. She lives in the adjacent neighborhood Buguruni. When Saada's husband realized the severity of his wife's illness, he sent word to her to come and take over.

Fellow tenants also help if somebody falls ill. They organize transport, lend money for treatment, give advice on treatment options and cook food for the family. In such emergencies, relatives and neighbors link up as informal security networks. They give moral and practical support, pool resources and help to master the situation.

5.2 Receiving and giving support

Receiving support

In the household interviews we asked about support not only within the household (Chapter 4.2) but also beyond the household. The open-ended questions were: "Who helps you apart from those you live with? When and how do they help you? Where do these people live? And why does this help assist you in improving the health of the household?" *(Mbali na unaoishi nao unaweza kupata wapi msaada? Msaada gani? Na wakati gani? Watu hawa wanaokupa msaada wanaishi wapi? Kwa nini msaada huu unakusaidia kuboresha afya nzuri nyumbani?)*

As listed in Table 18, our study participants mentioned various kinds of support which we assigned to our general categories of health activities.

Table 18
Receiving support beyond households (multiple answers)

Health activity	Relative	Neighbor	Total
Generating income	11	3	14
Providing food	31	13	44
Ensuring cleanliness	1	1	2
Taking care of children	17	8	25
Providing health care	6	4	10
No support			29
Total	66	29	124

Several women have received financial help from relatives. This kind of help ranges from occasional gifts to substantial support.

> When my brother visits, he gives his nephews money, and so does my father.

> My father's brother who lives in another part of town helps me a lot. He assisted me in finding a secondary school for my child and even pays her school fees. If I don't have money and ask him, he always helps me.

Neighbors sometimes help out with small sums, but they rarely provide continuous support over a long period.

Concerning food provision, women most frequently mention food gifts from relatives living in rural areas. When they visit the city, they bring food, either staples or specialties that are not available, or too expensive, in Dar es Salaam, for instance fish from Lake Nyasa or banana from Moshi or Morogoro. Some women or their relatives visit the rural areas, often at harvest time, and receive staples like maize, rice or millet.

> My husband's relatives have a *shamba* [field, garden] in Kibaha. They help me a lot because they bring rice, cassava and coconuts. They also grow vegetables that I cannot get at the market.

> Whenever relatives from my home area come to visit, they bring me food from the *shamba*, for instance cassava, fruit, maize and banana.

> When my relatives travel up country, they bring me food such as maize and beans. This adds to the nutritional value of our diet and helps us to use our money for other needs. They bring this food as gifts.

> I get help from my mother once a year. When I go home for a holiday, she gives me maize and beans.

If neighbors or friends travel, they may also bring back such food gifts. More often, however, women talk about another custom practiced among neighbors, namely the casual exchange of small items like salt, onions and sugar.

Only two women give examples that fall into the category of cleanliness. A young man occasionally fetches water by car. In one case, this man was a relative, in another case a neighbor.

The help listed as childcare reiterates what we discussed earlier. Relatives provide daycare, take over if the mother travels or raise foster children. Neighbors keep an eye on the children while the mother goes to the market or to town.

Concerning health care, relatives give advice and visit if somebody is ill. Two of these relatives work in hospitals. Neighbors also help to bring patients to the hospital.

It should be noted that women do not mention health activities organized along the principle of rotation *(zamu zamu)* or contribution *(kuchangia)*, namely paying water bills, cleaning the environment, disposing of garbage or emptying cesspits. These organizational principles do not fall under the category of help *(msaada)*.

Another interesting point is that a third of the women (N = 29) claim not to receive any help.

> Nowadays, it is not easy to get help even from your relatives because everyone is fighting against the harsh conditions of life *(kila mtu anapambana na hali ngumu ya maisha)*.

> Right now life is difficult. There is nobody helping another person. Everyone is to himself *(ninaongeza msingi wangu*, literally: I add to my own basis)*.

Four of these women live in single-parent households, the others in nuclear, polygamous, extended and even compound households. Their statements can be interpreted as expressions of vulnerability in the sense defined earlier (see Chapter 1.5). These women feel deprived of a social security network reaching beyond their own household. Whether their statements are objectively true is less important than the fact that they present themselves as lacking outside support from relatives and neighbors.

Four other women do not mention a relative, but a friend, a neighbor or an institution as a source of support.

> I don't have anyone apart from the mosque management. We get water free of charge and sometimes even clothes. The government used to help

us. They swept the roads and collected garbage. Now it no longer supports us.

This statement like others quoted in the preceding sections conveys a feeling of disappointment with the government. In this case, the mosque is mentioned as providing support. Other women refer to friends they meet in prayer groups or religious congregations.

> When we are sick, women from our church come to see us at the hospital. When I gave birth, they brought me presents, for instance soap, money, clothes and various other things.

Religious institutions and congregations replace, at least for some women, the social security network based on kinship.

Giving support

Every woman is, of course, not only a potential receiver but also a potential provider of support. For this reason, we asked the women still another set of questions: "What about help you give to people outside of the household? Do you give any help? What kind of help? To whom and when do you give this help? How does this help assist others in improving health?" (*Sasa kwa upande wako, je, wewe unatoa msaada gani kwa watu wengine mbali na kaya unayoishi nayo? Msaada gani? Kwa nani na wakati gani unatoa msaada? Msaada huu unamsaidiaje kuboresha afya nzuri?*)

We again classified their answers according to the list of health activities (see Table 19). We further differentiate between relatives and neighbors because we expect different rules governing these two types of social relationships.

Table 19
Giving support beyond households (multiple answers)

Health activities	Relative	Neighbor	Total
Generating income	32	–	32
Providing food	21	12	33
Ensuring cleanliness	1	–	1
Taking care of children	2	–	2
Providing health care	6	6	12
Other	9	4	13
No support			10
Total	71	22	103

The most frequent response to these questions was that women support their relatives by sending money, sugar and clothes, whether these relatives live in the same neighborhood, other parts of Dar es Salaam, another town or rural areas.

> I help the parents on both sides, my own parents and the parents of my husband. I send them money, rice, sugar and clothes at least once or twice a year.

> We have the responsibility of helping my husband's father and my mother's sisters. They are all in Tanga. When we get money, sugar or clothes, we send these things to them. You know rural life. If a person has money, sugar and some clothes, it helps very much because they cannot get them.

Some women also provide more regular and/or substantial support.

> My husband and I help my mother. We send her maize flour, rice and a sum of 2000 Tsh a month. The help assists her a lot because she is now old and cannot help herself. If we don't give her food and money, then her life is in danger.

> I help my mother. Our father passed away a long time ago, and my mother is still raising young children who go to school. I normally help my mother by paying their school fees. This gives our mother relief. She remains only with the responsibility of providing them with food.

> With me, all relatives depend on me, also my late sister's children in Bukoba. I help them with school fees and clothes.

A few women point out that they have taken in relatives to live with them. Others refer to help they give if a relative falls ill or gives birth.

With regard to neighbors, the most frequently mentioned kind of help is the daily exchange of small items like salt, onions and tea leaves. A few women recount how they helped neighbors when they had a life cycle ceremony.

A number of women (N = 10) report not being able to help anybody outside the household. Six of these women also claimed not to receive any help.

> I help no one. Life today means everybody to himself *(kila mtu anakwake).*

> I really don't give help to anyone because my own affairs are too much for me. How can I dare to help others?

> I am just what I am. I have nothing, as you see. I have neither front nor back. Hence, I don't give any help.

> I normally get helped. My situation is not all that good to enable me to help somebody else. I mean, I am not able to fulfill my family's needs.

It is possible that some women presented themselves as more vulnerable than they actually are because they expected us to mobilize some support from external sources. However, our personal impression was that most of these women lived in a particularly difficult situation.

Reconsidering reciprocity

To look more deeply into this issue, we focused on financial help. In an urban neighborhood like Ilala Ilala, an "ideology of assistance" is often, although by no means exclusively, formulated in financial terms:

> That's how we are. If a relative or another person who is close to you asks you for money, you cannot say no, even if you have only little to give.

How should we interpret such a statement? Does it mean that everyone helps everyone else? To answer these questions, we need to examine who receives what kind of help from whom under which circumstances.

The majority of the women in our sample (N=92) received gifts in the form of money *(msaada wa fedha)* at life cycle ceremonies, namely at marriage, birth and funerals, or in emergencies like severe illness.

> My husband's uncle gave me 5000 Tsh to make our wedding a success.
>
> At the birth of this child, my brothers gave me 3000 Tsh.
>
> When I lost my sister, my relatives gave me 1000 or 2000 Tsh in the form of incense *(ubani)* and shroud *(sanda)*.

Most women denote specific relatives from whom they received assistance. Some say, whoever has something to contribute gives some money. Still others mention relatives who form groups for such an occasion and contribute money, presents and labor, that is they help with cooking and looking after guests. Yet, not only relatives, also neighbors and friends are involved.

> When I lost my young brother, my neighbors and my parents-in-law came and brought me money and clothes.
>
> When I lost my sister, I got money and food as help from my relatives and friends.

What is remarkable is that the majority of the women (N=65) claim having received financial help only at these life cycle ceremonies.

Other women refer to specific relatives who provide financial help *(msaada wa fedha)* in certain situations, for instance in a sudden financial crisis, or for certain purposes, such as school fees, starting capital or the renovation of a house. We have already mentioned such examples earlier.

254

> In rare cases, my brothers give me such help, for instance when I am sick or broke.

> My parents help us when my husband gets stuck.

> We got such help from my husband's uncle and from my brothers. Our house was under renovation. Once we were short of money to buy equipment, so we had to seek money from them, and they gave it to us.

Obviously, some people do not have any close relatives who are able to help. Yet, even relatives who have financial means consider carefully to whom and to what extent they want to commit themselves.

> My husband's uncle has just returned from Saudi Arabia. We have tried to beg him to give us some capital, but he is still weighing whom he should help.

What is a typical feature of this kind of *msaada wa fedha* is that a repayment or counter gift is not expected. In this sense, we can speak of a "generalized reciprocity" (Sahlins 1965) which is often considered as a characteristic of kin relationships. "Generalized", however, does not mean that every relative will help just because he or she belongs to that social category. Women have to negotiate, and if they are lucky, they have a relative who is particularly committed to them or to a certain cause. We mentioned the example of a grandfather taking care of the special needs of a handicapped grandson. Another example is a father's brother providing practical and financial assistance for the secondary education of a child. On the other hand, such commitment seems to be commonly linked with kinship. Only two women in our sample said they could rely on financial help from close friends.

Another type of financial help is practiced more widely. Women refer to it as borrowing money *(kukopa fedha)*. The majority of the women in our sample regularly borrow small sums from relatives, neighbors, work mates or friends, but usually only from one or two persons.

> I borrow 100 or 200 Tsh from my brother in Lindi Street or from my neighbor.

> I borrow small sums like 100 Tsh from my neighbor, if I need money quickly.

This practice of borrowing implies a "balanced reciprocity" (Sahlins 1965), namely a direct or indirect repayment between two individuals on an equivalent scale. The currency of exchange may vary, but a balance has to be maintained. In other words, individuals may exchange services, goods and money with each other; the important thing is that they establish a pattern of ongoing mutual support acknowledged by both. If one gets too dependent on the other, conflicts arise and the relationship may be broken off. Apart from this continuous exchange, the women described two other practices, when we asked about *kukopa fedha*, namely buying on credit from shops (N = 24) and playing *upatu* (N = 19)[2]. Both practices are based on the principle of balanced reciprocity. While many women combine these types of "borrowing", others claim not to follow this practice at all (N = 28).

5.3 Discussion and conclusions

This chapter focused on the private-public interface of everyday health practice. The main question was how social dynamics shape women's response options regarding health activities reaching beyond the household into social groups, networks and institutions. Since we were interested in real rather than ideal behavior,

---

2   "To play *upatu*" is a local expression for participating in Rotating Saving and Credit Associations (ROSCAs). This institution has already been described for Dar es Salaam (Tripp 1989, 1992; Koda and Omari 1991: 123; Campbell et al. 1995: 239–240; Obrist van Eeuwijk and Mdungi 1995) and also exists in many other countries (Geertz 1962, Ardener 1964, Ardener and Burman 1995).

we first examined the social relations of health practice by scrutinizing specific task-centered interactions. In a second step, we systematically inquired into actual support, making an analytical distinction between "receiving" and "giving" support.

In principle, everyday health practice in Ilala Ilala is well organized, not only within but also beyond the household up to the government. During our main field research, the City Council was supposed to ensure garbage collection and other public services; the owner of a Swahili house was in charge of paying for these services; and the head of household had to contribute his share to bills.

This hierarchical system was, however, hardly functional. With regard to collection of solid and fluid waste, for instance, we found that City Council services were not reliable and favored households who paid extra fees and people with personal connections. Government representatives on the next lower levels – the ward, the branch and the ten–cell–units – knew about these problems and recommended residents, for instance, to dig garbage holes. They acted mainly as supervisors, while the house owners on the next lower level were responsible for implementing their advice. Most houses in Ilala Ilala were Swahili houses. Ideally, they functioned as corporate groups with reference to several health activities concerning all households, such as cleaning of communal facilities, water supply or garbage disposal. Households either provided equal contributions of labor (*zamu*) or money *(kuchangia)*. House owners were responsible for organizing the labor and collecting the money. In many cases, however, house owners only collected the rent and left it up to the tenants to organize themselves. Within the household, finally, responsibilities were divided between husband and wife. Cultural norms assigned "public" activities to men. In practice, much of the burden involved in these "male activities" had shifted to women. Men provided the money, while women were the main organizers. Since most husbands delegated their task to the wife, the weakest member – so to speak – ended up bearing the heaviest burden.

In the past five years, municipal governments took over from the City Council. They pushed privatization and sub-contracted various public services to companies. This and other measures have improved some of the services, for instance garbage collection and the provision with water for domestic use. They have not changed the social dynamics within the Swahili house and within households. Since women are usually most affected by and concerned about the negative effect of poor services, they end up playing the most active role in organizing these communal activities. One could argue that their engagement empowers women to take a more active role as citizens and members of urban communities, but this hardly reflects women's own view of the current situation. All in all, women emphasize negative aspects in terms of difficult tasks added to an already busy domestic agenda.

In conclusion, our data from Dar es Salaam confirm findings from Accra (McGranahan et al. 1996: 123–124). Poor households carry a heavier burden in terms of environmental health management than affluent households. They are forced to find their own solutions in terms of getting safe water, emptying septic tanks and disposing garbage, and this is not only a practical but also an intellectual challenge. Moreover, male household heads are the key decision-makers in terms of allocation of resources to support environmental improvement, while women bear the burden of environmental health management within the home (Songsore and McGranahan 1998), and we would add, at the interface between household, formal and informal services providers as well as social groups and networks.

We now turn to the second major theme in this chapter: receiving and giving support beyond the household. In general terms, an "ideology of assistance" (Lomnitz 1977) is also at play in Ilala Ilala. This set of values and rules allows people to mobilize a broad range of resources, a fact also described by previous researchers for other parts of Dar es Salaam. We argue, however, that this assistance is not given indiscriminately. For a deeper understanding of this core principle of social dynamics, we refer to a well-known analytical distinction in anthropology: generalized reciprocity and balanced reciprocity (Sahlins 1965).

Generalized reciprocity means that no repayment or counter gift is expected. It is mainly practiced among relatives, for instance if relatives collaborate in a small business or the husband's father provides vegetables from his field. What is often not sufficiently recognized is that even among relatives generalized reciprocity is an expression of a special commitment and bond, more particularly so if support is given regularly and/or over a long period. This is of particular relevance for a realistic assessment of kinship based response options. Our study participants receive help from and give help to specific relatives, and these are usually few in number. Moreover, they receive and give support in specific circumstances or for specific purposes. A certain brother, for instance, gives money to buy a sewing machine, so that his sister can start a small business, or a woman supports the children of her late sister.

Balanced reciprocity, on the other hand, implies a direct or indirect repayment between two individuals on an equivalent scale. This type of reciprocity is practiced between neighbors. Women who get along well exchange small sums of money, goods like onions, sugar and tea leaves, take turns in watching the children while the mother goes to the market and give assistance if somebody falls ill. In case the balance tips to one side because one woman asks for more than she returns, quarrels easily flare up.

In more general terms, our data clearly show that not only gender but also kinship relations have become subject to reinterpretation. While some women insist that generalized reciprocity is a kinship obligation *(wajibu kwa familia)*, the majority of our study participants consider it as "voluntary help" *(msaada)*. Moreover, in certain areas, the boundaries between relatives, neighbors, friends and work mates have become blurred, for instance in financial and practical assistance during a sudden crisis or at a life cycle ceremony. The social security networks of some women are based on social relations forged by religious faith rather than kinship. In other areas, though, the boundaries remain rigid. Only relatives take charge of a household, when the mother falls ill, or raise the children of parents who cannot take care of them.

A last and very crucial point is that the social cushion of many women is thin. The majority of our study participants (65 percent) report having received financial help only at life cycle ceremonies or in emergencies. Nearly a third asserted they do not receive any support outside the household, and a smaller group stated that they do not give help to others (10 percent). Illness, we have seen, is not only frequent among people living in such an environment, it further depletes already scarce financial and social resources. If women do not have relatives who are able and willing to help, and if they cannot engage in reciprocal exchange with those they live with, their situation may rapidly change from bad to worse.

6 Vulnerability to urban health risks

This chapter builds on the previous ones and suggests a framework for examining the links between urban health risks, response options and vulnerability on the household level. The leading question is why some women fare better, or worse, than others although they live in the same urban neighborhood and are exposed to similar health risks.

Our approach builds on previous studies on vulnerability (see Chapter 1). We examine the interplay of the "external" and the "internal" side of vulnerability. According to Chambers (1989: 1) the external side of vulnerability is characterized by risks, shocks and stress, while the internal side refers to "the lack of means to cope without damaging loss". The terms "risk" and "stress" imply that people are not necessarily exposed to sudden and unpredictable disasters but may have to contend with a range of forces that are constant and predictable (TzPPA 2002/03: 19). The main urban risks described by Moser (1998), commoditization, environmental hazards and social fragmentation, fall into the second category. Based on our discussion of urban development in Dar es Salaam, we suggest that these more constant and predictable threats combine with many uncertainties and contingencies resulting from an urban crisis, global change and structural reforms.

Our basic assumption is that vulnerability increases if women are confronted with more urban health risks and have less access to effective response options (see Figure 2). To compare exposure and responses to risks across households we draw on the approach developed by Krüger (1997). The main methodological difference is that we focus on individual women, not on households. In the next section, we select a few key response options identified in our study, arrange them along a continuum and classify the women

Figure 2
The interplay of urban health risks, response options and vulnerability (modified after TzPPA 2002/03: 18)

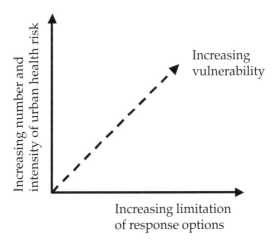

of our household sample (N = 100) according to whether their response options increased or reduced the urban health risks they were confronted with. We then narrow the focus on case studies from the cohort study (N = 20) for a close-up view of the dynamic dimension of vulnerability. Selecting a few women from each category, we follow their health practice over several months. This also enables us to gain a better understanding what "effectiveness" and "social acceptability" mean with regard to the response options in this particular local context.

The combined comparative and case study perspectives will show that women face a series of interrelated dilemmas which affect their vulnerability. This opens a new line of inquiry which can only be outlined in this study, namely a systematic examination of human agency in vulnerability. We introduce the concept of resilience to point to further directions in which this kind of research should develop.

6.1 Degrees of vulnerability

Based on the data presented and discussed in the previous chapters, we now select four key response options to urban health risks resulting in different degrees of vulnerability (see Figure 3): 1) applying public health knowledge to ensure cleanliness, 2) choosing between gender models, 3) mobilizing support within the household, 4) mobilizing support through social networks and groups.

In our study, women's health conceptions draw on health development discourses. Their statements emphasize in many different yet patterned ways the importance of basic needs, personal and household hygiene and care. To compare women across households, we focus on the application of public health knowledge in reported health activities. As a cut-off point for using/not using public health knowledge we decided on three activities.

Women's access to financial means is crucial for putting their health knowledge into practice. How they can gain access is to a large extent regulated by gender models. In the predominant gender model, a wife has the right to rely on the husband as main breadwinner and authority. In reality, however, many men were not able or willing to live up to this cultural expectation. Most women in our study sample (70 percent) began generating additional income and contributing to household provision. Probably in response to these changes in the household economy, several gender models have developed, and women have to choose between them. They either continue to rely on their husband, they generate their own income to contribute to household resources or they rely on their own means. Since women combine these options in different ways, we defined two indicators. Women either do or do not rely on financial support of the husband, and they do or do not generate their own income.

In an urban environment, where sanitary conditions are inadequate, reproductive work requires continuous efforts in the form of labor, time, money and intellectually capacity to sustain

Figure 3
Socially and culturally relevant response options

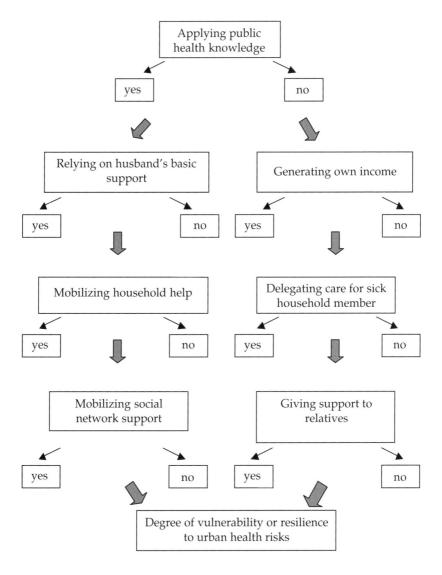

health. A crucial question thus is whether women succeed in organizing support from other members of the household. This becomes especially critical for women who pursue an income generating activity. Support is necessary for routine health activities like cooking, cleaning and child care. It becomes even more relevant, if a member of the household falls ill. As mentioned earlier, the burden of illness was high in our study sample. In nearly 70 percent of the households, one or more member(s) had been ill during the weeks prior to the household survey. The burden of reproductive work of course increases with the number of dependents living in a household. In the definition of indicators, we decided to distinguish between mobilizing household support for routine health activities and more specifically for health care. The cut off point was having more than four dependent members in the household and no person older than twelve to provide substantial help with reproductive work.

If governments fail to provide a healthy environment through adequate infrastructure and services, citizens have to mobilize many resources through social networks and informal groups. In Chapter 5, we investigated various interactions women have with persons beyond their household as they carry out specific health activities. Some of these activities such as cleaning communal facilities, disposing of garbage and emptying septic tanks are organized within the Swahili house community and link households with often informal service providers. In these conditions, it is a moral obligation to help relatives and sometimes even close friends, especially in times of crisis or for festivities marking a life cycle event like marriage, birth or funeral. People, in other words, do not only receive but give assistance, whether they consider it as an obligation or simply as help. Some women in our study sample even gave substantial and continuous support, for instance by paying school fees for younger siblings or by providing long term care for sick relatives. For this reason, we also defined two indicators for support through networks and groups: One option is to mobilize support, the other to provide support.

After identifying these key options and defining the indicators to "measure" them, we proceeded to classify each woman. For this purpose, we translated each option into a question yielding a "yes" or "no" answer. We asked, for instance: Does the woman follow the dominant gender model and fully rely on the husband for access to financial means? If the answer was "yes", we considered the response option as limited. According to our model, vulnerability increases if response options to urban health risks are limited. These indicators thus enabled us to clustered women into categories based on the degree of vulnerability. Those with only one or two negative answers formed the "least vulnerable" group, those with two or three "no" answers the middle group, and those with four or more limitations the "most vulnerable" group.

The "least vulnerable" group is the smallest (N=15). Five women in this group belong to the comparatively well-to-do Indian or Arab households; others have Bantu and/or Swahili backgrounds. They are well informed about the importance of household hygiene for health and put their knowledge into practice. These women make use of several effective options and live with one or the other risk: Some fully depend on their husband and do not work. Others spend much time in taking care of a sick member in the household. Still others do not receive any support through social networks or groups. Several women give support to relatives staying with them and consider this as a burden. All female household heads in our study confronted at least one additional risk and were thus classified as belonging to the middle group. Even though the women in this group are better off than the others, it is important to emphasize that they are potentially vulnerable. Risk factors quickly multiply in this urban neighborhood, as the next section will illustrate.

Most women in our sample belong to the middle group (N=58). Most of them apply some basic public health knowledge. Although many of them partly rely on their husbands, they are also involved in some productive work. Their income makes a difference, even if it means only a small increase in the daily budget. On the other hand, they suffer the double burden of productive and reproductive work, especially if they have not managed to enlist an adolescent or grown up person to share in the arduous tasks. Those who work longer hours, and away from home, usually earn more but, at the same time, suffer more if they do not have reliable support in daily health activities performed within the household. The burden of all women in this group increases if a household member falls ill and requires care. Substantial support given to a mother, sister, brother or another relative further depletes the resources of some women. Some women heading single-parent households earn a good salary but face the problems we just mentioned. All in all, the women in this middle group have more limited options and face several risks. They have little scope for managing critical life events or emergencies. As we shall see in the next section, some of them persevered and stayed on the same level, others hit a downward spiral.

Women of the third group (N = 27) are the most vulnerable because they have even fewer options. Some emphasize how difficult it is to apply their health knowledge. If they are married, their husbands commonly make irregular contributions to household expenses. Often, this combines with a lack of independent income or being overburdened with productive and reproductive work. Sickness and the resulting increase of risk in practical, emotional and financial terms is another common problem. Some women neither receive nor are able to give support beyond the household. The women in this third group are in existential difficulties. Any added risk may have severe consequences for the individual woman or the whole household. As we shall see in the case studies, some women managed to mobilize additional resources, others continued to live in this precarious situation.

One could, of course, read our model also reversely: Even under these difficult circumstances, most women have some space for decision and action. It is at this point that human agency comes into play in the study of vulnerability. We suggest that some women fare better under the same circumstances than others because they are able to use the same response options more effectively. From a salutogenic perspective (Antonovsky 1987), their ability is partly a result of general resistance resources like personality, physical disposition and micro-environment, partly an outcome of successful coping strategies. Human agency can hardly influence general resistance resources but it drives coping strategies. "Coping" is a fuzzy term defined in many different ways by many different people. We prefer the concept of resilience. In the strict sense of the term, we see "resilience" as the ability of a person to "bounce back" after being affected by negative influences resulting from urban health risks.[1] From a broader perspective also embraced in our study, resilience encompasses various ways of "coping" or successfully living with these risks. This rises the question what we mean by "successful". In our study, the most important criteria are that a person acts in a socially acceptable and effective way enhancing her sense of health and well-being. This may mean avoiding, resisting to, contending with or overcoming urban health risks. It certainly involves a weighting of response options and risks and a pro-active use of positively evaluated options.

Our research data suggest that we need to oscillate between vulnerability and resilience to best capture local experiences of health in everyday life. Each of them illuminates important dimensions of this construct which we call health.

---

1   This definition of the term resilience refers to its use in studies on different materials; they tested, for instance, how far a metal rod could be bent without breaking, and whether it would spring back into its original position (pers. com. Peter Nagel).

6.2 Dynamics of vulnerability

Case studies best capture the interplay of vulnerability and resilience. They will show that both concepts have to be understood as dynamic processes, not as unchanging states. Our findings, however, also suggest that the urban health crisis has pushed some women and their households beyond the point at which they can be resilient. If the burden grows too heavy and/or the decline is too rapid even the most resourceful women have to give up.

The least vulnerable group

Zuhura

Zuhura is a well educated woman with secondary education and a degree from a teacher's college. In addition to her formal job in Ilala Primary School, she employs a man to prepare and sell ice-cream. Her husband Ali is a clerk at the harbor, they are both Moslem, and she regards him as head of the household who leads the family. They not only raise their own four children but also a child Zuhura had with another man, two children of her sister-in-law and a child of her brother-in-law. Their home consists of two rooms in a Swahili house which Zuhura owns together with two brothers who also live there.

During the household interview in October 1995, we were impressed by the cleanliness and the family atmosphere in this house. The adolescent girls and boys, for instance, shared two separate bedrooms in the backyard. Zuhura's household was well organized, and she had much to say about domestic hygiene. The only risk factor to be detected in the interview data was the sickness of her niece Mwajuma. The girl suffered from TB and came to stay with them without explaining her problem (see Chapter 5.2).

On the first follow-up visit in March 1996, we found Zuhura pregnant. She now had a house help who, together with her fifteen-year-old daughter, supported her in daily health practice. Zuhura instructed and supervised them. What surprised us was that Zuhura kept her cooking oil in her room, not in the kitchen, and she locked the door of her rooms whenever she left the house.

When we visited her again in April, she told us about a conflict she had with a sister-in-law who lived in the same house. This woman, Amina, also participated in our cohort study (see below). According to Zuhura, Amina was jealous because two of Amina's children were mentally retarded, while her own children were bright and healthy. She accused Amina of estranging her brother to such an extent that their conflict had to be taken to court.

In May, Zuhura gave birth. She had sent away the house help and arranged for a trusted relative, namely the daughter of her sister-in-law on Ali's side who lived in Mwanza, to come and take care of her and the baby. Zuhura's children performed all the health activities under her supervision. Apparently, Zuhura had lost the court case against her brother. At the end of the month, they had already moved to another neighborhood.

The case of Zuhura illustrates that women can reduce their vulnerability through social ties within and beyond the household. Social relations however always mean potential conflict, and conflict often leads to increased risk. In this case, the conflict with her sister-in-law not only caused Zuhura emotional harm, it also added a financial burden and reduced the security of living in the house where she had grown up. Since we did not follow her into the new neighborhood, we do not know whether Zuhura fared better or worse in her new home. This first case study further draws attention to the importance of pregnancy, birth and infant care in women's lives. Zuhura was able to mobilize additional sources of support and did not suffer a loss of income because she received maternity benefits. For other women, getting pregnant and having a small baby become risk factors, as later case studies will show. All in all we conclude that although major changes occurred in Zuhura's life situation over the cohort study period, she remained in the least vulnerable group because she had an economic and social cushion and was able to make good arrangements.

Zuhura was committed to knowledge derived from public health and, perhaps because she was a teacher, she imparted this knowledge to her children and the house helper. Since she worked part time away from home, she delegated certain health activities to her children and the house helper. However, this did not have a negative effect on the quality of health practice because the household was well organized. Social interactions clearly influenced her decisions, not only in daily routine. As the date of birth was approaching, Zuhura made arrangements for her relative from Mwanza to come because she knew from previous experience that she could trust her. The decision to leave the family house was a result of the negative social interactions she had with her sister-in-law and of the court decision.

Rose

Rose is also a teacher and works in Ilala Primary School. To earn additional income, she gives tutorials at home. Over time, many parents have become convinced of the benefit of these tutorials. One hundred children attend, and Rose employs a second teacher. He takes over the morning sessions, Rose teaches in the late afternoon. Her husband William is a trainer in the army. They are both Christians, have seven children and rent two rooms in a Swahili house.

During the household interview in November 1995, Rose presented her conjugal life with William in terms of partnership. As parents, she said, they look after their children and take care of their health, education and life in general. Each of them contributed the salary to the household income. She further told us, William as well as the children helped her in daily health practice.

Her health explanations and descriptions of health activities were precise and detailed. Outside the household, she relied much on her mother who lived in Magomeni, another neighborhood of Dar es Salaam. Rose did not have to provide substantial support for anyone. She gave the usual presents at life cycle ceremonies or in emergencies, and once a year she sent money to her relatives in Morogoro. Based on this interview, it seemed that Rose did not face any of the risks we looked at.

During the follow-up visits in March and April 1996, Rose was always very busy. During the day, she taught at the primary school. She came home, had a shower, changed clothes, ate something and started the evening tutorial. Her children did all the house work according to a schedule. Rose gave instructions and supervised them, when she had time, for instance on weekends.

It was only during the fourth visit that we learnt Rose was running a *de facto* female-headed household. A year ago, William had been sent to Arusha, a town in Northern Tanzania. Since it was a special military training, the men were not allowed to visit their families. At least she received half of his salary.

At the end of May, during our last visit, she confided it was high time for William to come back. She was so busy earning money, had hardly any time for her seven children, and they needed a strong hand to guide them. When she was at work, they often did not follow her instructions. Especially the nearly one-year-old baby was not always cared for properly.

Rose had the knowledge and commitment to reach the highest standard of nutrition, hygiene and child care possible in this neighborhood environment. To put it into practice, she did her best to provide the financial means and to instruct and supervise her children who carried out most health activities. Her husband normally supported her, not only with his salary, but also in taking over some of the house work and guiding the children. However, the longer her husband was absent, the more her vulnerability increased. Rose moved from the "least vulnerable" towards the "middle group" in the course of the cohort study because several risk factors had increased: she received only half the salary from her husband, she lacked his support in the household which also influenced the reliability of the support she received from her children, and nobody beyond the household assisted her in managing her daily life.

Her interactions with the children influenced decisions regarding the daily routine, for instance the allocation of tasks or instructions regarding child care. Even her absent husband had an impact on her decisions and course of action. She worked harder to earn enough money and had less time for the household, the children and herself. Her emotional distress increased, and it is well possible that she took measures to improve her situation soon after the cohort study.

Joyce

Joyce has a high school education and an accountant diploma. She does not work in her profession but earns an independent income by raising chicken in another neighborhood of Dar es Salaam. Her husband Nelson is working as a car mechanic, they are both Christians, and they raise three children in two rented rooms in a Swahili house.

During the household interview in December 1995, Joyce was well informed about health matters. She regarded careful planning as essential for ensuring health, her household was organized, and her rooms looked very clean. Although she seemed self-assured, she considered Nelson as head of the household because he was her husband. With his salary, he was able to provide more than adequately for the daily household needs, and she contributed only to special expenses. When she had the last baby, they arranged for the child of one of Nelson's brothers to live with them. Victor was a boy of twelve years, and he helped Joyce with child minding and other health activities in the house. Her husband also supported her in house work and took care of buying staple food in large quantities because he had access to a car. In terms of external support, she did not face the burden of giving substantial help to anybody, except for the usual presents. The only risk we detected was that she claimed not to have anybody to support her outside the household. Her husband, in fact, did not like her to mix with the neighbors. All in all, Joyce was happy and full of plans. She was well situated and owned many appliances such as a music system, gas cooker, fan, television set and fridge.

On our first follow-up visit in March 1996, we found her selling ice-cream to school children. This money, she said, allowed her to buy soda for her children or guests whenever her husband was not around. Some people came to buy boiled water she kept in the fridge. Joyce quickly calculated that the money she earned from this activity would cover the electricity bills. She further told us Nelson had left for South Africa to buy two cars which he would then sell in Dar es Salaam. He had called her the other day saying he had reached the Zambia-Tanzania border. However, he was delayed by some problems with documents and would be back in about ten days.

In mid-March, Nelson was not yet back. Joyce looked tired and worried. Two of her children had a fever, and she suspected it was malaria. She wrote down an exact description of the symptoms and sent Victor to a pharmacy run by a European woman. A street vendor passed with water, but he asked for Tsh 150 per container, and Joyce wanted to pay only Tsh 100. She complained she needed water to do the laundry. She then carefully prepared lunch, fed the baby separately, put the children to rest and sat down with Victor to watch television.

On the third visit, we first only met Victor carrying the baby. When Joyce arrived, she looked stressed. After taking care of the baby and instructing Victor, she joined us and said her budget was exhausted. Nelson was still not back. She had heard from a friend of her husband that one of the cars he had bought in South Africa had probably been stolen. The engine number did not correspond with the number on the car documents. The customs officers had confiscated the car, and Nelson was back in South Africa to either procure the proper documents or to reclaim his money. It was now four months since he had left Dar es Salaam, and the money he had given her for household expenses was used up. Joyce now bought the daily food with the money she earned from her chicken project.

When we asked whom she could turn to for support, she said, the only person was the twin brother of Nelson. He was selling second-hand clothes at Kariakoo market. After three months, he had stopped visiting her. When she went to see him at his stall, he said he would hear no more of her problems because he had no money to give her. She then went to Nelson's father's brother in another neighborhood of Dar es Salaam, but he was away for some months. Her neighbors, she asserted, were already talking behind her back, and, the other day, the house owner came to inquire about her plans for the two rooms.

We inquired what she would do if her husband stayed away for some more weeks. Would she earn enough from her chicken project to feed her family? She replied that, during the past weeks, she had had to sell the chicken in order to buy food. One possibility was to sell beans at Kariakoo market. If she had some capital, she could go to her home village in Morogoro and buy beans in large quantities, perhaps 10 or 20 kilograms. One of her uncles would help her with transport because he worked as bus driver on the route Morogoro-Dar es Salaam. Another possibility, she said, was to approach her aunt. She owned a big farm on the outskirts of the city and was looking for someone to market her passion fruit. Joyce thought she could make a good profit if she managed to sell the fruit to the big hotels in the city center. We encouraged her to follow-up on this possibility.

On our next visit, we again found the home in disorder. These days, Joyce was so busy looking for money, she had hardly time for her children and the domestic tasks. When we met her, she told us about her activities of the past few days. To save money, she left early in the morning, walked all the way to her aunt's farm, picked up some passion fruit, carried them back to the city and sold them to the beverage manager of the Hotel Excelsior. She had impressed him with her story, and he had agreed to help her. The money she earned allowed her to buy food. While we were chatting, her eldest son came running and asked Joyce for empty beer bottles. She told Victor to fetch them. A man walked in and offered Tsh 60 per bottle. Joyce bargained for Tsh 100, but the man insisted on Tsh 60. Joyce replied she would sell him only fifty bottles for that price. They finally agreed on Tsh 80, and he carried the bottles away. She turned to us and said: "See, that's how bad it is. I even have to sell beer bottles, and now none are left. At least I can now buy the baby's milk which costs Tsh 80 per day."

On our final visit, Joyce had given up her passion fruit business because it was too tiring and the profits too small. She was depressed, started crying and asked us for help.[2] We agreed to give her a loan to start the business with the beans from Morogoro. In the following weeks, she often stopped at our house to report about the ups and downs. All in all, she had managed to stabilize her situation, even though Nelson had not yet returned.

This case study demonstrates how rapidly one risk factor leads to another and vulnerability increases. When the financial contribution the husband had left was used up, Joyce quickly exhausted the resources which had enabled her to gain an additional income. She could no longer take sufficient care of health sustaining activities, and the house helper was too young to take full charge on his own. She concentrated her energy on earning enough money to feed the family. When her children fell ill, her meager resources were further depleted. Still, she ingeniously found ways of earning a few shillings here and there. One of her relatives supported her for some time, but then his means and/

2   Although this was a research project, not an intervention, we had put aside some money to help women in dire straits, especially those who actively participated in our study like Joyce.

or willingness came to an end. Other relatives were prepared to assist only in initiatives leading towards economic self-reliance. Since she had not invested in good relations with her neighbors while she was doing well, they kept their distance and did not offer any help. Although she struggled hard, Joyce moved from the "least vulnerable" to the "most vulnerable" group in the course of the cohort study because she lacked the financial and social means to overcome her problems. Without our help, she might not have been able to stabilize her situation.

The case study further illustrates that many decisions Joyce took were influenced by direct or indirect interactions with others. The problems she faced were the result of her husband's difficulties at customs. It was also her husband who had advised her not to mix with the neighbors when she was still well cared for. Although she was strongly committed to follow public health messages, she could not do so because she had to concentrate on earning money and lacked reliable support within the household. Whether she could save a few shillings on water or earn some money depended on her negotiations with the water seller, the man who bought beer bottles, the beverage manager in the hotel and her relatives.

Fatuma

Fatuma has a primary school education and pursues three income-generating activities at home: She keeps ducks, employs a tailor and sells second-hand clothes. Her husband Hamisi drives a public bus. Both of them are Muslim. They raise three children of their own and three children Hamisi had with another woman. Hamisi's mother, brother and a child of this brother live in the same household. They occupy two rooms of a Swahili house owned by Hamisi.

During the household interview, Fatuma referred to Hamisi as head of household. According to her, male headship is part of the cultural heritage, but men actually depend on the advice of their wife, and the household is led by the woman. Fatuma had basic health knowledge and tried to put it into practice, although not wholeheartedly. She seemed rather ambivalent, for instance when she remarked that human beings could not clean water, while water cleans them. Her husband provided adequately for household expenses. Her mother-in-law had a farm, her father-in-law an income from renting out rooms, and both of them occasionally contributed to the household. Fatuma helped her brother and her sister in times of need but not on a long-term basis. The only risk we could discern in the interview data was that Fatuma had to take care of her children when they were ill.

On our first follow-up visit, we found the mother-in-law resting on a mat together with the small children. Fatuma was lucky since she had not only her mother-in-law but also other women to support her, namely a house helper who did most of the cleaning and assisted in child care, and her younger sister. Fatuma's sister was actually staying with them because she had malaria. She sold cold water to earn a few shillings and helped with household chores. Regarding business activities, Fatuma told us that nearly all ducks had died. She now mainly relied on the trade in second-hand clothes. Her biggest worry was the brother-in-law who was staying with them. He had chased away his wife and was now using bad language towards Fatuma and his mother.

On the second visit, another old woman was in the household. We learnt she was the mother who gave birth to Hamisi. The other grandmother who permanently lived in Fatuma's household and cared for her children was his step-mother. The real grandmother had come because Fatuma's daughter Zawadi had to be hospitalized.

When we came back the next time, Zawadi had recovered. Fatuma's younger sister was still staying in their household. When we arrived, she was cooking the main family meal. Fatuma told us life was becoming increasingly difficult. She now had only one iron, the other one had been stolen. We learnt that it is not she who trades in second-hand clothes, she rather provided the facilities for male traders to wash and iron clothes. With only one iron available, the queue grew long, and some of the traders started to look for other facilities. As Fatuma further recounted, she had begged her husband to make his brother leave. This brother and the children were a burden since they depended on Hamisi's income and Fatuma's services. However, her husband thought it would be difficult to make them go.

When we paid her the last visit, Fatuma proudly showed us the small tailor workshop she had set up on the verandah. Also, she had rearranged their rooms to make space for a storage facility. She now rented out this new facility for Tsh 300 per day.

This story again documents that many of our study participants were preoccupied with earning money. Fatuma was particularly skillful in creating new opportunities without leaving the home. She was much less interested in child care and domestic work and delegated most of these tasks to other women. Since she was actively involved in a continuous exchange with several relatives, she could always find somebody to support her in reproductive work. On the other hand, her case illustrates that support to relatives becomes a burden, if relations are not balanced in one way or another. Although we discovered another risk in Fatuma's life situation, namely the continuous and substantial support given to the brother-in-law and his children, and although she was confronted with illness during the cohort study, Fatuma had been able to raise additional financial and social resources and thus remained in the "least vulnerable group".

Again we see a woman interacting and negotiating with others. Fatuma took charge of her life as much as she could but her decisions and the course of actions she took depended to a considerable degree on the people she lived with. Since she was more committed to earning money than to housework and child care, she gladly left these tasks to other women and was fortunate to have their support. Her husband obviously agreed to the initiatives she took, except for her plea to ask his brother to leave.

The middle group

Amina

Amina is the sister-in-law of Zuhura (see above). She has a primary school education and does embroidery as an income generating activity. Her husband Hassan works as a clerk in the City Council of Dar es Salaam. Both of them are Muslim. They raise four children of their own. Two grown-up sons of Hassan and one of his younger brothers live with them. They have two rooms in the Swahili house owned jointly by Hassan, another brother and Zuhura.

During the household interview in October 1995, Amina discussed health activities in detail and emphasized that she closely observed each point in daily practice. She considered Hassan to be the head of household because of his ability to have a formal job and to provide adequately for his household. Amina performed nearly all health activities herself. The young men occasionally assisted her in washing and ironing clothes and sometimes went to the market. Outside the household, she said, neighbors helped her when she needed them. Relatives occasionally brought presents, and she assisted them in times of illness. All in all, she seemed well situated and embedded in a social network. The risks we noted were that she had to do most of the house work herself, and her husband as well as her child had been ill recently.

On our follow-up visits in March 1996, Amina told us she neither trusts food vendors nor water vendors in terms of hygiene. She would rather walk all the way to the market to buy fresh food and fetch water either in the flats across Uhuru Street or in a nearby hotel. Amina assured us that she always boils the drinking water. She wondered whether it was really worth the effort. She and her children may have to drink unboiled water if they visit neighbors, and catch diarrhea. She was weighing the risks and clearly enjoyed discussing them.

On our fourth visit, we learnt Amina had stopped doing embroideries. She did not go into details, but it seemed well possible that she would later pick it up again, since she had practiced this handicraft since she got married in 1982. Amina was very busy with her two mentally retarded children. Very patiently, she taught them simple domestic tasks. We never saw her interact with neighbors or visitors. She kept very much to herself and never mentioned her quarrel with Zuhura to us.

As this case study shows, women who are not or only marginally involved in earning an income have much more time for reproductive work. This enables them to increase their control over health practice, especially if they are committed to ensure hygiene. Amina was committed, and she tried her best to impart her knowledge to the children, although they were mentally handicapped. Still, they remain exposed to risks in the neighborhood. A potential danger for Amina and her household was her apparent social isolation. When we last saw her, she depended completely on her husband and had hardly any social interaction beyond her household. Perhaps this problem was solved after her sister-in-law moved out of the house. In general, her risk of vulnerability had neither increased nor decreased during our cohort study.

Nuru

Nuru has not been to school and earns an income as a food vendor. Her husband Juma is already in his sixties and has retired from his job as a clerk in a glass factory. Both of them are Muslim. They have five children and rent one room in a Swahili house.

During the household interview in November 1995, Nuru explained she shared headship with Juma. He gave her a lump sum to pay for water and electricity bills and the rent. She then budgeted the remaining money for household expenses, but it was never enough. She always had to contribute. Nuru had clear ideas about health and what was needed to sustain it. Her twelve-year-old daughter Asha supported her in putting them into practice. Just a few days before the interview, her two youngest children had been ill, and she had to take care of them. Then, as in life in general, nobody helped her outside the household. Her own support for others was restricted to occasional presents. The impression we had after the interview was that Nuru was a hardworking, charming and welcoming woman who faced three risks, namely inadequate household provision by the husband, lack of support beyond the household and sickness.

When we met her again on the first follow-up visit, she sat on a mat outside the house with her little daughter on her lap. Next to them was a tray with pasta she had put there to dry. She asked us to sit down and told us about the illness of her daughter, and the worry it caused her. Since she had spent all night in hospital, she had not been able to prepare food for her business, and without income from her business, she was unable to pay the Tsh 1000 for the Chloroquine syrup prescribed for the child.

On the second visit, she had just got back from Bodi, the place where she sold her food. Nuru had an exceptional daily routine. She got up at 2 a.m. to cook pasta and rice pies. At 5.30 a.m., she left the house to walk to Bodi. Her husband and her fourteen-year-old son Imamu accompanied her and helped her carry the pots. Around 10 a.m., they returned home and took a nap. Nuru then did the cleaning and prepared the main family meal. In the afternoon, she went to the market to buy rice, took it home to clean it and then brought it to the milling machine to grind it into flour. Imamu often helped her by going to the milling machine, while her husband Juma walked to the factory to buy the pasta.

On our third visit in April, a neighbor guided us to Nuru's room. She was lying on the floor on a piece of cloth. When she saw us, she tried to sit up but was too weak. She was suffering from malaria and had had her last injection the night before. There was a knock on the door, and a fellow tenant brought some food. Nuru saw it was *ugali* (maize porridge) and *dagaa* (small dried fish) and said she did not feel like eating. The woman carried the plate away. A sick person, Nuru explained to us, needed good, nutritious food to go with strong medicine like Chloroquine, for instance fruit, green vegetables and meat-broth, not "food for hard times" *(chakula cha shida)* like maize porridge and fish. We said she should tell her husband to bring her good food, but she only laughed. "Juma," she replied, "has many words in his mouth but no money in his pocket." She then became serious and confided she was deeply worried. There had been so much illness in her family lately, perhaps it was the modern disease (AIDS). She had even discussed it with her sister who worked in the laboratory of Muhimbili Hospital. Now, she really was at the end of her strength and without her income, her family could not survive. Most probably, she would move in with her mother in Kipawa. One of her children already lived there, the other one was staying with her sister.

When we went to look for her the next time, the neighbors told us she had moved. Some weeks later, she came to our house to tell us that she had left her husband because she would be better off on her own. Her smaller children were staying with her mother.

This case study shows again how rapidly risks increase and cumulate, pushing people into an existential crisis. The fact that Nuru had fostered out some of her children indicates that she was in a precarious situation even before this crisis. Her financial, emotional and physical resources were further depleted when first her children and then she herself fell ill. Perhaps Nuru already belonged to the most vulnerable group at the time of the household interview. The additional risk and the lack of support in managing it caused the household to dissolve.

Although Nuru would have liked to ensure cleanliness and child care, she was hardly able to do so due to economic constraints. All members of the household had to contribute to her business because it was the only way to fulfill at least the most basic needs. Nuru dedicated all her time and energy to this most basic health activity. Since the interactions with her husband increased rather than decreased her financial, practical and emotional burden, she decided first to move to her mother's home and then to separate.

Anna

Anna is the head of a single-parent household. She has a primary education and works as a secretary, has three children and a house helper. They live in two rooms of a Swahili house.

During the household interview in November 1995, Anna discussed various aspects of health and complained how difficult it was to improve health "if you have to crack your brains for basic needs such as food". Still, she had a steady income, could afford a house helper and always looked well groomed. Other people, she said, did not help her, not even the father of the children. She sometimes sent money to her mother in Mbeya. Although Anna seemed comparatively successful and aspiring to move up in society, we noted three risks: She did not have a husband to share the burden of household provision, nobody beyond the household seemed to support her, and one of her children had been ill.

When we first went back to see Anna in March 1996, we were surprised to find her at home at ten o'clock in the morning. We assumed she was sick, but she told us she had decided to stay home because her house helper had lost a relative and took leave to attend the funeral. Anna said she did not feel like fetching water all the way from Chunya or Mtwara Street. When a water vendor passed, she called out to him and began bargaining for a good price.

Anna was still at home at the end of March. She looked uncomfortable and unkempt. As soon as we joined her, she told us about a fellow tenant who had fallen severely ill during the night. When she saw a woman who lived a few houses further down the street walking towards the house to visit the patient, Anna asked us to move inside. She said she was not on good terms with this woman. Just because she was an Arab and her partner had money she thought she could say anything. She had told all the women along the street that Anna had lost her job. She even advised the women who played *upatu* with Anna to exclude her immediately, otherwise they would have to run after their money.

We asked whether she had quitted her job. Anna replied, it was not yet confirmed. She had not received her salary for three months because the government had no money. She thus decided to stay home until she got her wages. Her plan was to start a small business, and she actually was expecting her sister to visit her to discuss this matter. Soon afterwards, her sister arrived by car. She carried a big box, and Anna asked us to join them as they went into her sitting-room. Her sister traveled to Zaire and Sambia to buy cloth which she then sells in Dar es Salaam. A three-piece *kitenge* fetches up to Tsh 23'000. These *vitenge* (Singular: *kitenge*, plural: *vitenge*) were very popular. Women liked to wear them to weddings and other celebrations. Anna would get Tsh 2000 from her sister for each *kitenge* she sold. Her sister encouraged her to take up this business.

On our fourth visit at the end of April, we saw Anna sitting all by herself with the little daughter on her lap. The other tenant women were chatting on the other side of the house. As we passed them, they said we should rescue Anna because she was facing hard times. When we joined Anna, her little daughter was crying. Anna explained the other women had asked their children not to play with her children. In fact, a fellow tenant whom she considered her friend had slapped her daughter because she wanted to drink tea with the other children.

After a while, her daughter fell asleep, and Anna carried her to her bedroom. She came back with two letters. One of them informed her of her dismissal, in the other one, the worker's committee asked her to contribute Tsh 2000 to bring their demands to court. Anna said she did not have the money because the children were going without food. The other day, she received Tsh 5000 from a friend, now she did not know whom else to ask. Her sister might give her another loan at the end of the month, if she could afford it. Since January, Anna had begged money here and there because she was waiting for her salary. Until now, the government had not handed out any money. If she could work for our research project, she would do anything we asked for, even if it meant counting all the people in Ilala. The debts she now had were almost as high as the outstanding wages, and people refused to give her any more loans.

The next time we met Anna, she was bargaining with a butcher through the shop window. She looked better than during our last visit. As we walked towards the house, she told us she had gone to her office and had been promised the outstanding salary and allowance until the end of the month. She could now resume her life. If she asked people like the butcher for a loan, they would once again agree to give it because soon she would be able to settle her debts. When we arrived at her house, she went straight to the backyard and entered a small shack. The house owner had ordered her out of her rooms.

After changing her clothes, Anna joined us, and we sat down in the backyard. When she saw her little daughter come out of the toilet, she nearly cried. She said, she felt ashamed seeing her children walking barefoot, especially when they entered places like the toilet, but there was nothing she could do about it. She had tried to communicate with the father of the children but, until now, he had not shown up.

This case study demonstrates how hard the Civil Service Reform hit low-level clerks who were dismissed in large numbers. As long as friends, neighbors, and shop-keepers believed Anna would sometime in the near future receive the money the government owed her, they agreed to give her money and goods on credit. However, this type of exchange was clearly based on "balanced reciprocity" (Sahlins 1965). Even fellow tenants who used to be her friends, and especially women who enjoyed neighborhood intrigues, cut her off from these exchange relationships when she could no longer reciprocate. Anna received help *(msaada)* in the form of general reciprocity from her sister. Yet again we find that relatives provide such support only for a certain period and not in amounts substantial enough to cover all household expenses. They then switch to a different mode of support, namely encouragement and practical help in initiatives leading to economic self-reliance. Within the household, Anna lost the assistance of her house helper because she could no longer afford to keep her. Even without an illness in the household, Anna's vulnerability had rapidly increased during our cohort study, and she moved from the "middle" to the "most vulnerable group".

Anna had been committed to keeping her children in good health, but when she lost her job, she could no longer afford to do so, and this caused her emotional distress. Moreover, since she was used to being formally employed, it was difficult for her to earn an income in the informal sector. Anna not only lacked the skills of a business woman, she probably did not put all her energy into this kind of activity, even when it was offered by her sister, because her mind and heart were fixed on receiving the outstanding salaries and allowances. She felt cheated by the government, and this blocked her initiative. Her decisions were to a large extent influenced by her interactions with government officials. What further influenced her course of action were her negotiations with people she asked for credit. That the father of her children as well as her neighbors did not provide any support was most likely the result of previous interactions.

Victoria

Victoria is also the head of a single-parent household. She has a secondary education, a diploma as an office management secretary and works in the state house. In addition to her own three children, she cares for two children of her brother and a child of her late sister. They live in two rooms of a Swahili house.

In the household interview in December 1995, Victoria had much to say about health. Her household was well organized, and she received support from adolescent daughters as well as from a house helper she employed. The father of her youngest child occasionally assisted her, and she gave the usual presents to her mother. All in all, Victoria seemed capable of managing her household. The two risks we observed were that she did not have a husband to provide regular support and no assistance beyond the household.

When we arrived for our first follow-up visit, Victoria was not yet home from the office. One of her daughters asked the other one to get the boy ready, as Victoria would soon be home. The second girl picked up the boy, bathed him with soap, changed his clothes and put him to bed. When Victoria arrived, she first asked the girls whether Tomasino was asleep. She then went to her room, came back with a *khanga*, had a shower and changed her clothes. Soon afterwards, the father of Tomasino arrived. She introduced him and told us they were going to get married the next month. Victoria frankly told us she longed for married life. He was a member of her church, and she trusted him. The father of her first and second child refused to marry and went out with other women. She thus had decided to leave him and to rent two rooms in Ilala Ilala on her own.

During the next visit, we spent most of the time with the adolescent daughters. They did the laundry, cooked, fed Tomasino, bathed him and changed his clothes. They put him to bed for a nap, invited some school friends for lunch and had a rest. When Victoria came home from work, she took charge and inquired closely what they had done.

We planned the next visit for a weekend and found Victoria very busy. She had just returned from shopping at the market and complained that the girls had not cleaned up the dishes before they left for their tutorials. She unpacked ripe bananas, oranges, fried fish, green peas and corn cobs. While we chatted, she prepared the fruit and invited us to join her in a light meal. This was her lunch, she explained. Like many people in town, she skipped a meal whenever possible. Since the children would spend their day in tutorials, she would only prepare one hot meal in the evening.

Life had become really difficult, she told us. Since neither her brother nor her late sister had any money, she raised some of their children and paid for their education. Back in the 1970s, nobody would have thought of starting a small business, but since 1993, she earned some additional money by making popcorn. She had bought six kilograms of corn cobs, because a work-mate had placed a special order for her daughter's birthday party. Usually, Victoria packed the popcorn into small plastic bags and sold them in her office for 50 Tsh each or in two shops along Uhuru Street for Tsh 40 each; the shop-keeper took Tsh 10 per bag in commission.

On another weekend, Victoria was in the kitchen and was boiling the drinking water for the coming week. She explained she did not trust the girls when it came to this task. It was also Victoria who allowed us to visit when the local experts came to empty the cesspit.

During our last visit, she instructed her daughter to clean "the environment". She said, the two older girls were responsible, but she wanted her younger daughter to learn each household task. It was important to teach and supervise adolescent girls. Only then would they learn to carry out their responsibilities properly. She had also instructed the older girls when they came to live with her. Sometimes, she threatened to send them back, for instance when they left Tomasino playing in muddy water outside the house. "When you come across a little boy on the street with bare feet and dirty clothes, it drives you mad! But if the mother does not take care of her own children, no one else will do so."

As this case study shows, Victoria was quite successful in managing her household, even though she had a full time job and a sideline activity. In many ways, she was privileged, especially in comparison to her brother and sister, and for this reason she felt obliged to help them by raising and educating some of their children. However, as she herself said, it was difficult to do everything on her own. If she fell seriously ill or lost her job, she would soon face the same risks as some other women in the neighborhood. To get married to a responsible husband would enable her to reduce this risk, but by the end of May, her wedding plans had been postponed. All in all, Victoria remained in the middle group throughout our cohort study because she continuously faced two risks, namely no husband to support her and giving substantial and long-term help to relatives.

Victoria was obviously committed to household health, although her time at home was limited. Since she was in charge and knew that adolescent girls are not yet fully responsible, she decided to be strict and to guide them with a strong hand. Her example further underlines that decisions which involve other people, like getting married, have to be negotiated. Having an independent and relatively substantial income enabled her to leave the fathers of her first two children without suffering a damaging loss when she was not able to reach an agreement.

The most vulnerable group

Sada

Sada went to high school but did not finish it because she failed her exams. She does not have an income generating activity and lives in a polygamous household. Her husband Salim sells potato chips. Both of them are Muslim. They have five sons and raise the youngest sister of Salim who has just started primary school. Sada and her children live in two rooms of a Swahili house, and her husband takes turns staying with her and his first wife.

During the household interview in October 1995, Sada was well informed regarding public health messages. Her husband went to the market himself and left her some pocket money for small expenses. She considered him to be the head; he had taken her away from home and she did not have an income generating activity. Her young sister-in-law helped her with health activities within the household. Beyond the household, she said, nobody helped her. Shortly before the interview, her ten-month-old son had been ill. According to our classification, this added up to five risks, namely no independent income, no substantial support within the household, giving support to a sick household member and no help beyond the household.

On the first follow-up visit, Sada told us she had lived in this house since 1984. Water had become increasingly scarce. This made life difficult because water was needed for many purposes. As we talked, the children came back from fetching water. Even the three-year-old boy carried a pot.

Sada was usually engaged in some domestic task when we came to visit her. She either cleaned "the environment", washed clothes, kept an eye on the small children, cooked and tried to keep her rooms in order. What bothered her were the flies which entered the room from the backyard. She tried to kill them with insect spray but was not able to control them.

In mid-April, Sada fell ill with malaria and had to be hospitalized for five days. During this period, her sister living in the adjacent neighborhood took charge of the household. When Sada came back from hospital, her husband supported her in house work, even in cooking. We remarked that he took good care of his wife. He seemed happy to hear that and explained many men did not really know what was written in the Koran. Women were weak creatures. It was best for them to stay indoors, and the only duty they had was to bear children. Women should be well cared for, and the husband should pay for whatever work they did in the home. Yet that did not mean husbands should not do any house work.

During this and subsequent visits, the main worry Sada had was the difficulty of keeping children clean. Once, when she saw us off, she found the young boys playing in a pool of dirty water. They ran away when they saw her, and she shouted at them. She then went to fetch a hoe and tried to open a small channel to drain the pool. The hole was too deep, and the rain continued to fill it up.

This case study illustrates how women can persevere, even in a precarious life situation. Sada's husband fulfilled his responsibility to her and apparently also to his first wife, not only in terms of financial support but also in terms of caring and practical support. Sada performed most health activities herself, and the boys helped her occasionally. When she fell ill, her sister took over. In other words, her life situation neither improved nor changed for the worse, even though she passed through a severe illness, because she had a safety net which protected her from existential crisis.

Sada said she was committed to keeping her family in good health, but she often failed to do so and attributed her failure mainly to the neighborhood environment. Although it worried her, she seemed to have resigned and entrusted the children's health at least partly to God. Many of her daily decisions were influenced by her interactions with her husband. She not only depended on him financially, he also took a close interest in domestic work and child care.

Sakinah

Sakinah has no formal education. She bakes flat bread *(chapati)* as an income generating activity. Her husband is employed as a taxi driver. Both of them are Muslim, and they live with four children in a rented room of a Swahili house.

During the household interview in January 1996, Sakinah seemed less informed regarding health matters than most women in our sample. She explained these were issues for those who had been to school. Her husband went to the market every day, and she added to daily expenses from her own income. She considered him as the head because, as she put it, "he is the one who keeps us in town". Her eldest daughter was nine years old, and

Sakinah did all the house work herself. Beyond the household, nobody helped her, and her youngest child had been ill. Sakinah faced, in other words, five risk factors: She had little public health knowledge, her husband did not provide adequately, she did not have substantial support in the household but had to care for a sick child, and she lacked assistance beyond the household.

When we arrived for the first follow-up visit, she was cooking in the backyard. It was Ramadhan. She said the prices of beans had increased suddenly from Tsh 250 per kilogram in December to Tsh 400 in January. This was due to the increased demand; one of the main dishes to break the fast was made of beans. She had to stop preparing *chapati* because she could not sell them during the day, whilst people were fasting. Sakinah further told us her son Sultani suffered from sickle-cell disease and had to attend a clinic in Muhimbili Hospital every three months. She had lost her first son to this disease and now feared for her second-born.

On our next visit in April, we asked about the sick boy. Sakinah said they had decided he would be better off with his grandmother in Temeke (see Chapter 5.2). While we were there, she continued with the household chores, swept the room, the corridor and the courtyard, washed the dishes and chatted with the fellow tenants. They all scooped the water from a large container. Salma left one of the cooking pots on the ground to soak and carried the other dishes back to the room. When she returned, she saw one of the ducks she keeps in the backyard drinking from the pot, but she remained indifferent. Sakinah then got ready to do the laundry and sent her son for some soap. The first bar he brought was too expensive (see Chapter 3.3). She separated her own clothes from those of her husband and children because she suffered from a skin disease.

We arranged for Sultani to see a doctor who had agreed to provide medical help to the women in our study. According to his diagnosis, Sultani did not suffer from sickle-cell disease but from malaria, probably with a complication of hepatitis. He asked Sakinah to bring Sultani for a second test, but throughout our study, she did not return. The boy went back to stay with his grandmother.

On our next visit at the end of April, Sakinah asked us to go outside the gate, so we could talk. As we sat there, some neighbors passed and asked whether Sakinah had visited their friend who had given birth. Sakinah replied she did not want to go empty-handed. This friend had brought her a dozen new baby nappies and five liters of cooking oil when she gave birth to the now three-year-old Rahma. Perhaps next month she would have money to buy a gift and visit her friend.

When the women had left, Sakinah told us the entire household now depended on her income from *chapati*. In January, her husband had lost his job as the owner of the taxi had sold the car. Until now, he had not found any other employment. She now got up at midnight to bake more *chapati* than before, but she could only secure the capital for the next day's business and buy beans or maize flour. She said it was a secret in the house, and we should not tell anyone in the area. They planned to go back to Pemba Island because life had become too expensive in town. Her parents had promised her a plot to build a local house on, and they would grow cassava for the family. Luckily, her husband had paid an annual rent last year, and they still had three months to go.

This is another case showing the risk of dependence on one main breadwinner. Sakinah had an additional income, but it did not suffice, especially in a household already exposed to many other risks. The prolonged sickness of her first son had depleted her savings, and the long illness of the second-born had further strained her budget. Even though Sakinah could foster out her sick boy to her mother-in-law, the existential crisis deepened. Mobilizing additional social resources, she made first arrangements to solve the crisis by moving back to her home village.

Sakinah's decisions in daily health practice were not only influenced by her lack of knowledge but also by the economic constraints she faced. In interaction with her husband and mother-in-law, she had decided that her sick child would receive better

care in the household of his grandmother. She had further negotiated with her mother about her plan to move back home.
Whether her husband agreed to this decision was not clear. The
house owner, the fellow tenants and her neighbors were not supposed to know, probably because Sakinah feared their reaction.
To move back home would mean to admit failure.

Pili

Pili is a widow. She has not completed primary school and earns
her living by frying fish. She lives with five children in a room of
a Swahili house.

During our household interview in October 1995, Pili mentioned several aspects of health derived from public health knowledge. Her fifteen-year-old daughter and the younger children
helped her with the house work. She could not assist anyone beyond the household and had received substantial help from her
married daughters. Two of her children had been ill in the weeks
prior to the interview. Pili, in other words, faced four risk factors:
lack of provision by a husband, inability to help others beyond
the household, need of support from people beyond her household, and an additional burden of caring for sick children.

When we arrived for the first follow-up visit, Pili was frying
fish and chatting with a friend. At the same time, she was
breastfeeding her youngest child. When she got up to look after
the fish, Salum started to cry. She decided to wash him down
right where we were and then put him to bed in her bedroom.

Pili later told us, she did not want any more children. The
father of Salum had only given her his office number. He was
already married, used to visit her twice a week and had once left
her Tsh 10'000 to 30'000. They had got along well, and he had
promised to set her up in another house. When Pili got pregnant
with Salum, he visited her and told her he had problems with his
wife. Apparently, the wife suspected him of having an affair and
threatened to leave him. He had promised to visit Pili again in a

few days, but he never did. Pili called him at his office, and all he said was she should continue the life she had had before they met. She saw him again after the birth of the child. Because she had lost much weight, he thought she had AIDS, and he never came back. It was a very hard time because Pili and all those who knew her thought she had AIDS. Her married daughter supported her, although she did not have much herself, and gradually Pili recovered. Since then, she had stopped having affairs.

On the second visit, Pili wanted to discuss family planning methods. There was obviously a new man in Pili's life, either for pleasure or for securing a livelihood. She worked very hard and did not rest on weekends because she needed the money. She told us she could not even afford to buy an exercise book of Tsh 250 for her daughter.

When we met again, Pili looked young and beautiful. She was eager to tell us she had resumed dating. That day, she was not in a hurry and had enough money to buy Salum an ice-cream. She said she normally takes a day off to clean the house and do the laundry.

In the following weeks, however, Pili went back to her usual routine and never mentioned dating again. She spent all her time on fish selling and had hardly any time for domestic work and child care. We rarely saw her children except for Salum. Pili usually cooked one hot meal in the evening and warmed up the leftovers for breakfast.

This case study shows how difficult it is for a woman with a small income to raise children on her own. Three of Pili's children went to school, and she could hardly raise the money for school fees. Any extra costs were an additional worry. This left little time and energy for reproductive work, and nobody was there to help her. This case further illustrates the special vulnerability of women caused by their reproductive ability, both in terms of having children and maintaining the household. Pili's life situation was precarious and did not change in the course of our cohort study. At the beginning it seemed as if she might be able to improve her living condition with the help of a new partner, but this help, if it ever existed, was only a short relief.

The story of Pili shows that she invests all her time and energy into the most basic health activity, namely to ensure livelihood. Like many other women, she had once decided to improve her life by becoming the mistress of a comparatively well-to-do man. He left her when she got pregnant and did not take care of her when she was ill. This past interaction had influenced Pili's course of action for the next two years. She did not get involved with any man. When she considered this option again, she wanted to protect herself by joining the family planning program. She did not carry out the decision, perhaps because most clinics demand to see the woman and her partner.

Christina

Christina has a secondary education and does not earn an income. Her husband Ernest is a business man. Both of them are Christians, and they live with three children in one room of a Swahili house.

During the household interview in December 1995, Christina was knowledgeable about health matters. Her husband was not able to provide adequately, but she considered him as the head. Her eldest child was an eight-year-old boy, and Christina performed all health activities herself. She sometimes received presents from a member of her church, and she could only give spiritual help to others. Nobody had been sick recently in her household. We thus counted four risks: inadequate household provision by the husband, no independent income, no reliable support within the household, and inability to give practical or financial help to others.

During the first follow-up visit, Christina looked unhappy. Her family had been moved from the main house to a single room in the backyard. She was busy doing the laundry; it had rained during the night, and they were able to fill all containers.

Christina and Ernest have lived in this neighborhood for a long time. They had been much better off. She worked in a bank until her husband told her to quit because he earned a good salary as senior clerk in the headquarters of British Petroleum (BP). However, two years ago, he was dismissed, and since then they have had a very difficult life.

The next time we visited her, she had just come back from fetching water in another street. A middle-aged woman joined us and went to Christina's room. Christina explained, this woman had been suffering from what many people would call AIDS. She had actually been possessed by bad spirits. Since Christina convinced her to join her church, the woman felt much better. To show her gratitude, she came to assist Christina with cleaning and child care.

The two women quickly prepared a hot meal because they were planning to attend a special prayer meeting which would be held daily for the next nine days. While the pots were on the charcoal stove, the women washed the children and dressed them up. Christina then had a shower and prepared herself. After the meal they left in a hurry.

When we came to see her again, she was giving her room a thorough cleaning. They had heard some mice during the night. When her son came back from school, he eagerly joined his mother in the mouse hunt. They managed to kill a mouse, but Christina complained that would not help much because there were many more around. Her husband was the one who really knew how to get rid of mice.

On another day we found Christina praying with a man. She said they did so every Tuesday and Thursday, rotating from one house to another to spread the word of God. The man, she explained, had been possessed by evil spirits. He suffered for a whole year and even lost his job. After he joined her church, the power of God had healed him.

Christina explained that she did not have much time these days to take care of the house work and of the children because she allotted as much time as possible to God and the Christian mission. When she still worked in the bank, she had a house helper, but now she could not afford one. For a while, she had been bogged down with all this work like most women in the neighborhood. Since she had joined this church, life had become much easier for her. Sometimes, her husband ironed the clothes for the whole family; sometimes another Christian woman came to assist her as we had seen the other day. All this, she said, was a blessing of God because the other women had no time for any other activities and for their spiritual life.

Christina's story is about a woman who suffered a shock two years ago when her husband lost his job and has gone though a rapid decline of her living standards, which also entailed humiliation. She found comfort in a charismatic Christian church, and this also enabled her to mobilize social resources. During the cohort study, she faced additional difficulties, such as having to move to the backyard, but her overall life situation did not change with regard to the risk factors we examined.

Although Christina had sufficient health knowledge, she opted to invest her time and energy in religious activities rather than in health activities. She entrusted her own and her children's health primarily to God, although she visited a hospital when her young daughter suffered from diarrhea. Most decisions in her daily life are influenced by her faith and by the people with whom she interacts in her church.

6.3 Interrelated dilemmas

The discussion of these case studies clearly demonstrates that women face a series of interrelated dilemmas. They have to choose between interrelated options, and some of these options present an opportunity as well as a constraint. We consider this point essential for a better understanding of human agency in vulnerability. To underline it we reconsider some of these dilemmas, and add some evidence from previous chapters and field notes.

Concerning the first option, applying basic public health knowledge, the conventional assumption is that this knowledge presents a resource that enables women to make their homes a healthier place. In this view, health knowledge only becomes a risk factor, if it is not available and/or not accurate. Our data suggest, however, that in a situation of delayed medicalization, as we observe it in Dar es Salaam, public health knowledge itself becomes a risk: It may cause emotional distress, especially for those women who have accepted it as a code of values and rules, but cannot put it into practice. This comes out once again in these case studies, and additional evidence has been presented earlier (Chapter 3).

To rely on the husband's financial support is – as most women have insisted – the culturally defined right of a wife. In this sense it is a positive option, as long as this support is adequate. It is obvious to all that well cared for wives can take better control of household health practice. On the other hand, women learn from their own experience that complete dependence on the husband often turns into a risk. Even if the husband is willing and able to assume responsibility, he is likely to be absent for an extended period, lose the job, fall ill or even die. Such a sudden change commonly leads to an existential crisis because money circulates and is hardly ever saved.[3] Women are aware of this risk; some more than others, particularly those who stopped their income

---

3   In such circumstances, the rotating credit and saving associations *(upatu)* which are rather popular also among the women in our household sample do not provide a safety net. As explained in more detail elsewhere (Obrist van Eeuwijk and Mdungi 1995), the purpose of these *upatu*-groups is not to save money for difficult days. Women join these groups in order to separate small amounts of money from the daily household budget. By taking this money out of daily circulation and contributing a share (e.g. Tsh 100) to a common pot, women enable each other to get access to a slightly bigger amount of money once in a while, namely when it is their turn to

generating activities, for instance when they gave birth to twins, lost a child or had a health problem. These examples illustrate once again the interconnection of reproductive and productive work in women's lives.

Earning an income is a new, although contested, value and competes with women's main responsibility for reproductive work, not only in intellectual but also in practical terms. Our data clearly show that women's productive work affects the quality of health practice unless she can mobilize household help. Most women are aware of this link but still more are preoccupied with earning an income to complement the husband's allowance. If money is scarce and budgets are tight, any contribution makes a difference. The loss of a job opportunity, even if it was an informal arrangement, has a damaging effect, for instance in the case of a food vendor whose stall was destroyed during a City Council campaign to clean the environment (see Chapter 5.1). Such a loss is, of course, even more severe if the woman is the main breadwinner of the household, as the case studies of Nuru and Anna have shown. The case studies have further demonstrated that, important as they are, women's incomes in the informal sector were generally too low to adequately cover household expenses. Much better off were women who had a job in the formal sector because it guaranteed a steady income and special benefits, for instance maternity leave. However, since employees may be dismissed, the safest way for women was to combine a job in the formal sector with a sideline activity in the informal sector.

---

receive the collected money. If eight women play *upatu* once a week, each of them receives Tsh 800 once in a period of two months. If kept in the household budget, the money would have been "eaten up". Even though the amount women receive on a rotational basis is small (Tsh 500 = US $ 1). It allows them to make a purchase they could not otherwise afford. This system cannot help a woman to overcome an existential crisis because she actually contributes as much as she eventually receives. Moreover, as the case study of Anna has shown, women who cannot afford to make regular contributions may be excluded.

301

Social support is another complex value and creates much ambivalence in women's lives. To emphasize this often neglected issue and in order to allow for a more detailed analysis, we integrated this ambivalence into our definition of response options and examined receiving and giving support, both within and beyond the household (see Figure 3).

Whether women receive reliable support within the household partly depends on biological factors, namely the age and sex of their children, and partly on cultural and social factors, that is on whether women educate their children in the proper performance of health activities. Most women pass the prevailing gender model on to the children and concentrate their training efforts in domestic tasks on daughters, as we have seen in the case of Victoria. Several women emphasized that their husbands assisted them by guiding the children with a strong hand, or wished him to do so. To have responsible and well-trained daughters is an enabling factor because it gives women time and energy for other activities. If children are too young or overburdened, however, their involvement in house work becomes a risk factor.

Giving support and care to members of the household is an important aspect of women's gender identity (see Chapter 2.2). This encompasses, of course, most health activities, and especially the care for children,[4] but in this chapter we focused on their responsibility to care for sick household members. Especially minor childhood illnesses, as we have seen, are managed within the

---

4   Many women know from experience that giving birth to, and caring for, many children requires more strength than having only few children. Family planning was a topic in several household interviews and came up again in the cohort study. Several women reported practicing family planning, and other women would have liked to do so but lacked access to family planning programs for various reasons. Our study focused on the household maintenance dimension of reproductive health, but these findings indicate what many studies have advocated, namely that safe contraceptive methods contribute to reducing the vulnerability of women and their dependents (Harcourt 1997, Pollard and Hyatt 1999).

household, and most women first seek health care from biomedical facilities (see Chapter 4.1). This practice helps to reduce physical vulnerability. At the same time, it incurs considerable costs. Many women mentioned that sickness quickly depletes financial, social and emotional resources, and this becomes an even heavier burden if children suffer from a chronic illness, as illustrated by the case of Sakinah.

Support beyond the household becomes particularly relevant in emergencies, which are, unfortunately, common in such an environment. Most women relied primarily on single-stranded networks, for instance on a female relative on their own or the husband's side, to help them if they fall ill or give birth. The case of Fatuma who lived in a family house and was embedded in a multi-stranded network of relatives was the exception rather than the rule, even though many people described such an arrangement as the typical Swahili household. The secretary of the CCM branch in Ilala Ilala (see Chapter 2.3) confirmed that this household model was rapidly disappearing because relatives who inherited a house often sold it. They did so either due to family conflicts or in order to raise money for their own household. In our sample, most households were based on a nuclear family, confirming that family structures and underlying values are changing.

In this chapter, we focused on prolonged and substantial support and found that relatives provide such support only for a limited period of time. They then switch the mode of assistance and provide moral and practical support for the dependent relative to become economically self-reliant. What Obbo (1981: 117) has described for Kampala in Uganda also applies to Dar es Salaam: Nothing is free in town, and urban life has taught people economic self-reliance in spite of continuing ethnic and kinship obligations. This shows again that not only gender but also kinship values and rules are currently subject to reinterpretation.

Several case studies have further illustrated the importance of reciprocity in social relations, not only between relatives but also between neighbors and, in a different form, between members of voluntary associations based on ethnicity or religion. Members of Moslem as well as Christian congregations emphasized the importance of these relations of mutual moral and practical support. To invest in social relations is a critical factor for avoiding isolation in times of need. "Living well with people", as one woman put it, has moral as well as practical value.

This leads to the last factor, namely providing care for relatives who do not live in the same household. Women are well aware of the fact that mutual visiting and the exchange of gifts, even if carried out only once a year, keep relationships alive and increase the probability of receiving help in times of need. This rule operates between relatives who live far apart. Geographical proximity calls for more regular contacts. However, extended caring for relatives is acceptable, as long as a balance is maintained. To take in adolescent daughters of a sister or a brother incurs costs, especially if they attend school, but their household help balances the relationship. If, however, a brother-in-law moves in with his children and "does not live well" with the other members of the household, he is soon considered a burden. Especially women who are comparatively better off frequently have to give substantial and prolonged support to relatives. In all these situations, the skill of providing assistance without damaging loss becomes an enabling factor.

This discussion has shown that our model of socially and culturally relevant options (see Figure 3) visualizes women's dilemmas. On the horizontal level, options can have either positive or negative outcomes with regard to vulnerability. If read vertically, we see that options interact synergistically and reinforce each other. To make the situation even more complex, many values and rules which underlie these options are affected by economic, social and cultural change. This creates a complex network of opportunities and constraints within which women have to develop their perspectives. To find an effective and socially acceptable course of action under such circumstances is not easy.

Our evidence suggests that in view of these dilemmas "ambivalence coupled with pragmatism" (Lock and Kaufert 1998b: 2) is often the most resilient response.

6.4 Discussion and conclusions

As indicated in this chapter, everyone experiences potentially harming risks or stresses. However, even when people face comparable hardships, they are not equally affected since individual men, women and children have differential resources to tackle them. In our sample, nearly all women have been affected by urban health risks. Differences between the "most vulnerable", "middle" and "least vulnerable" group are small and fluid. Moreover, most women experienced minor or major changes in vulnerability during the cohort study. Unfortunately, most of the changes we recorded caused more constraints than opportunities and pushed women from "least vulnerable" towards "most vulnerable", not in the other direction.

This chapter raised several points concerning methodology. In hindsight we see that our classification of households has been biased by the technique we used to identify them. Household interviews capture only the contours of everyday practice. Only in-depth case studies make the picture come to life. This is partly due to the fact that only few comparable studies exist for African cities, so that research has an exploratory character and cannot build on and refine existing data on health and vulnerability. Furthermore, regular contact over an extended period of time establishes closer relationships than a short visit for a household interview. Women may also protect their privacy and prefer not to tell a stranger about a conflict with a sister-in-law or the prolonged absence of the husband and the consequences this has for domestic health. Trust is a prerequisite for deeper insights into people's lives and takes time to grow. Still other aspects are self-evident to the interview and not worth mentioning, like for instance the support of the daughter in fetching water. These considerations mirror the general experience that practice-oriented research cannot be based on interviews in an artificial situation; it has to be grounded in spontaneous conversations and observations in the flow of daily life.

A second methodological point concerns indicators. Qualitative approaches highlight and contextualize local practice, and we all know that numbers are crude indicators for complex concepts and reality. Once our understanding of the complicated links of urban health risks, vulnerability and response options has improved and deepened, however, we should try to develop quantitative indicators which enable us to compare and to search for differentials within and between individuals and groups. Our model is a first step in this direction. We still have to work on the definition of these indicators, systematically investigate the range from most to least, rank them and add scores. In the future, such a health practice vulnerability index might be useful for the study of discrepancies and distributions, not of health risk but of response options.

In this chapter we tried to systematically relate urban health risks, vulnerability and resilience. We found that the three characteristics of urban vulnerability described by Moser (1998: 4) clearly manifest themselves in the day-to-day life of these and the other women in our study sample. The commoditization of goods and services forces many women to become preoccupied with earning an income. The hazards of the natural and economic environment make emergencies like illness, death, loss of job or business failure a rather common occurrence. Even if a person is fortunate and does not face a crisis in her own household, these situations are part of her social experience as relatives, neighbors or work mates go through difficult times. Social fragmentation shows itself in the fact that women interact with only few other inhabitants of the same neighborhood.

This last point is of particular interest to us. As several case studies have shown, most women have single-stranded relationships with relatives who live in other parts of Dar es Salaam or even in rural areas. Women often have little knowledge about and trust in fellow tenants and neighbors and hardly participate in the social life within the neighborhood. They have of course daily interactions with fellow tenants, if they live in a Swahili house, and they meet people when they go to the market or fetch water. Yet this does not automatically mean that they are on close, intimate terms with them. Some women become friends, visit each other and help each other out wherever they can. Others live like a large family, even if they are not related to one another, and a minority still lives in a Swahili family house and has multi-stranded relationships with relatives in Ilala Ilala and other neighborhoods. Most commonly, however, the women in our study sample create close personal relationships selectively, even with relatives, and their often single-stranded relationships reach into other neighborhoods, towns and rural areas and have to be actively maintained.

To help others in need is a moral obligation but, in real life, assistance is often limited due to various constraints in terms of money, time and geographical as well as social distance. These findings have been confirmed by studies in other cities which document that the permanence of social capital cannot be taken for granted (Moser 1998: 13). As long as people cope, they help others, but once their assets are depleted, they cease to support other people. The result is a mixed picture of erosion and consolidation of social capital under difficult economic circumstance.

What is important to emphasize is that these economic changes influence, but do not determine cultural and social values. As old values become contested and new ones are not yet firmly established, individual persons as moral subjects search for their own position toward this growing diversity within and between codes of conduct. It is against this background that women's struggle for health has to be interpreted.

Vulnerability to urban health risks clearly has a dynamic nature. Even if our methodology may have magnified them, several rather dramatic changes in women's lives occurred during the relatively short period of eight months between the first household interviews and the last follow-up visits: Nuru fell seriously ill and her family broke apart, Anna and Sakina's husbands lost their jobs and the return of Joyce's husband was delayed. In the household interviews, many women reported similar experiences in the recent past, and we can assume that several women not included in the follow-up study have been confronted with an existential crisis in the subsequent eight months. Emergencies like sickness, death or loss of income occur frequently, and this is the very reason why women emphasize the importance of cultural and social values like mutual help and reciprocity within and beyond households.

For all these reasons, we suggest adding a dimension to Moser's characterization of urban vulnerability: contingency. Women are exposed not only to continuous hardship but to unpredictable life situations, often caused by rapid changes. This is a fact of life in an urban environment, where morbidity and mortality rates are high and job security in the informal and formal sector hardly exists. The approach we developed based on the work of Krüger (1997) is well suited to investigate health practice in such a situation because it captures the dilemmas women face. Moreover, it does not simply investigate the relationship between risks and options or assets but brings the links between vulnerability and resilience into sharper focus. Vulnerability cannot be reduced by options, only by effective and socially acceptable use of these options, and this is what we mean by resilience. Both vulnerability and resilience refer to instability and processes, not to stability and state.

This means that a better understanding of the complex relationship of vulnerability and resilience may show us a direction for mitigating urban health risks. Our empirical data exemplify that women who can combine enabling factors are obviously at an advantage in terms of reducing vulnerability. Ideally, a woman marries a responsible husband providing adequately for household expenses, she qualifies for a job in the formal sector, sets up a sideline activity, trains daughters and house helpers in domestic skills and childcare to support her in reproductive work and finds a balance between receiving and giving help to relatives, neighbors, work mates and fellow members of voluntary organizations. Few women in Ilala Ilala match this ideal, but those women in our sample who fulfilled many of these criteria seemed best equipped to deal with the contingencies of an urban environment. We suggest that a resource-oriented approach to improve health and reduce vulnerability could take this ideal as a backdrop against which various alternatives could be developed, for instance in participatory research with women.

7 Health, vulnerability and resilience

7.1 Health

The first argument of this study is that health, as a positive and discrete notion, constitutes a fascinating field for anthropological inquiry. Health for us is a comprehensive concept closely linked to bodily, material, spiritual and social well-being, but what health means in a given locality is open for empirical research.

Up to now, medical anthropology, especially in the United States, has investigated a broad range of topics relating to illness and health care, from preventing disease to restoring health, considering local contexts as well as broad political and economic forces, all of them resulting in health problems. As one of the most innovative and rapidly expanding sub-disciplines, it made major methodological and theoretical contributions to anthropology as well as to various strands of cultural and social theory. However, as Massé (1995) rightly contended, it has neglected health as a positive reference ("référent" in French).

The first systematic approach to medical anthropology developed by Arthur Kleinman (1980) has become widely accepted. It focuses on concrete cases of illness and examines what signs people recognize and define as symptoms of illness (meanings), how they explain the cause of the illness (etiology) and what they do for its treatment (care seeking). A basic assumption is that these dimensions of an illness experience are systematically interrelated. Another and related idea is that the sick person and/or his or her care givers interpret this experience within broader frameworks available in a given society. These frameworks of interpreting illness constitute discrete and often even competing social fields, especially in a time of medical pluralism and globalization.

Our study builds on this approach but widens the perspective. We also focus on concrete persons and study what they think and do in times of illness, but we are even more interested in investigating how they define positive notions of health (health definitions), how they explain causes of health (health explanations) and what they do to sustain health (health activities).

For the investigation of these positive notions of health we draw on the work of anthropologists, social psychologists and sociologists in Europe, especially by Claudine Herzlich (1969) in France and more recently by Toni Faltermaier (1994, 1998) in Germany. Following Herzlich we contend that social representations of what makes a person healthy are distinct from those of what makes people ill. We are aware that such an approach, for analytical purposes, draws a sharper distinction between health and illness than exists in people's everyday experience, but our aim is to correct an existing bias that emphasizes disease, illness and health care. To underline this contention, we advocate an anthropology of health encompassiung anthropolgical inquiries into health *and* illness.

We propose that health as an embodied experience is universal but has not necessarily always been conceptualized as an experience bounded *by* the body. One could even argue that a concept of health which is primarily defined with reference to the human body is a unique invention of European culture and does not have conceptual correlates in cultures with other historical roots. Over the past centuries and decades, however, other understandings of health defining locally specific sets of knowledge and practice have been deeply affected by fundamental social and cultural transformations of colonial rule and, more recently, of health development and globalization. As anthropologists have documented for even the most remote parts of the world, local experience of illness is now intepreted and explained with reference to various frameworks, including the biomedical model. What has commonly received less notice is that the same transformations have also facilitated the spread of public health discourses through various institutional arangements, as Burke (1996) has shown for Zimbabwe and Manderson (1996) for colonial Malaya.

Our study in Dar es Salaam, Tanzania, provides additional evidence for the spread, and the local appropriation, of public health discourses as frameworks of interpreting experiences of body and mind. When we asked women about "good health" *(afya nzuri)*, they drew on various frameworks: On broader understandings of health and well-being in Bantu as well as Christian and Islamic religious thought, represented, for instance, by ideas such as *uzima* (vitality, life force) and *amani* (peace), but also on health development discourses, for example in statements emphasizing hygiene *(usafi)* and basic needs *(mahitaji muhimu)*.

Similar to Herzlich (1969) and Faltermaier (1994, 1998) in Europe, we found that women in Dar es Salaam are able to formulate not only discrete but multidimensional concepts of good health *(afya nzuri)*. In their health definitions they considered the condition of the body *(hali ya kimwili)*, whether it was portly, strong and looking well, and the condition of the mind *(hali ya kifikira)*, looking for signs such as joy, vitality and peace. Their health explanations linked conditions of the body and mind with specific living conditions *(hali ya maisha)* such as the fulfillment of basic needs, hygiene and care. In their descriptions of health activities, they referred to five major and related themes: generating income, providing nutritious food, ensuring cleanliness, taking care of children and providing health care. All in all, women used many words and phrases they had learnt from health development discourses as well as from public health messages, for instance *mahitaji muhimu* (basic needs), *chakula bora* (nutritious food), *kula vyakula machanganyiko mara tatu* (to eat a range of foods three times a day), *maji safi* (safe water), and *kuchemsha maji ya kunywa* (to boil drinking water). Their understanding of these terms and phrases often remains fuzzy and does not fully correspond with public health knowledge from which it was derived. Public health knowledge was reinterpreted in the local context and thus appropriated, not simply "adhered to" or "complied with", as expected by many health professionals.

Contrary to our expectations, study participants did not articulate humoral notions rooted in Arabic medicine, as reported by Swartz (1991) for Mombasa. We explain these findings by the fact that Dar es Salaam is a comparatively young Swahili city that was founded in 1862 and soon became a colonial capital, first under German (1884–1914) and then under British (1914–1961) rule. It is a city where cultural traditions which used to be historically separate became enmeshed, namely Oriental, Occidental and African traditions. The Swahili culture which emerged can be seen as a Creole culture marked by heterogeneity and diversity. Already in colonial times, missionaries and, later, government officials and civic groups imparted basic knowledge on hygiene, nutrition and sanitation (Beck 1981), and these efforts were intensified after Independence in 1961. The socialist government under the late President Nyerere regarded health as an integral part of development. In this context we quoted the mass mobilization campaign *Mtu ni Afya* (Man is Health) as an example. These ideas were further reinforced when hygiene came to be considered as an integral part of *mambo ya maendeleo* (development issues) (Fiedler 1983: 12). In the process, health education messages linking cleanliness with health have become embedded in broader discourses on domestic skills, Christian virtues, discipline, progress and modernity. These discourses have been spread through various media and institutions and reinterpreted in the light of new trends in health development. Over the decades, they firmly established the responsibility for domestic health as an integral part of female gender identity.

Since the participants in our study saw us as somehow connected with a health project *(mradi ya afya)*, they may have consciously or unconsciously overemphasized their public health and development orientation. Our explicit research interest in domestic health ("health in the home", *afya nyumbani)* possibly further enforced this orientation and led women to think more about certain aspects and understandings of health than about others. Still, the evidence presented in our study clearly shows that these women have access to, and command of, basic public health knowledge which they appropriate to meet their demands in everyday life.

We propose that a focus on local appropriations of public health and health development discourses is well suited for research in cities. It is not a coincidence that "public health" as a discipline originated in cities (Wohl 1983, Ashton 1991). The growth of cities leads to enormous problems of water supply, sewerage and garbage removal, especially under conditions of economic constraints and/or weak governance.

Various anthropologists have emphasized that a patient-centered view should be complemented by an examination of power relations shaping the spread and institutionalization of biomedicine, public health and health development. These include, for instance, critical medical anthropologists (Singer and Baer 1995, Baer et al. 2003) and proponents of social suffering (Kleinman et al. 1997). Especially efforts related to health as a public good, namely when they are destined to reach also the poorer segments of society, are always politically contested and call for a political economy perspective.

While we agree with their critique of a narrow focus on patients, we prefer theoretical perspectives emphasizing practice and agency. By doing so, we also modify the social psychology approach of Herzlich, Faltermaier and others mentioned above. Inspired by Michel Foucault (1963), Pierre Bourdieu (1977) and Anthony Giddens (1984) we move beyond social constructivism and focus on the dialectic relationship between social conditions as well as structural constraints, on the one hand, and people as individual subjects and social actors, on the other. In our study of health in Dar es Salaam, we found such a dialectic approach particularly useful because it is an urban setting marked by rapid economic and political reforms, social and cultural heterogeneity, diversity and flexibility. A practice approach forces us, on the one hand, to investigate these structural conditions which, on the other hand force people to find their own ways of sustaining and restoring health.

For a closer examination of structural constraints, we identified four broader forces shaping urban health risks, namely the environment, the economy, the government and the society, and reconsidered them with a specific focus on Dar es Salaam and Ilala Ilala, the study site. Our main finding here was that, in only four decades, citizens had moved from a period of great hope and major achievements in the 1960s through an austere crisis in the 1980s to rapid economic and political reforms since the 1990s. While the macro-economy shows signs of recovery, many reforms have had a negative cumulative effect on households, especially among low-income workers. It is hardly surprising that an absence of trust in the government, and, sometimes, even a lack of hope, are sentiments expressed by many citizens, not only in Ilala Ilala and similar neighborhoods of Dar es Salaam but in many parts of the Tanzania (TzPPA2002/03, Fjeldstad 2004).

We conclude that "medicalization" in Dar es Salaam has only been partial, or delayed, and puts especially women into a paradox situation. They know what they should do, but they do not have the means and capacities to put this knowledge into practice, for instance when it comes to the boiling of drinking water to kill germs (see also TzPPA 2002/03: 95). The same is probably true of most women living in similarly situated communities.

These findings are highly relevant for policies and interventions. Contrary to the widely held stereotype view, women in low-income urban communities do have basic public health knowledge. In fact, they are often exposed to too much and contradictory health information. To support them in their daily struggle for health, we should provide them not with more but with more appropriate public health knowledge from trusted sources and with the basic services that enable them to put this knowledge into practice.

7.2 Vulnerability

The second argument of our study is that the concept vulnerability best captures what urban citizens in Africa consider as detrimental to health and well-being. They are less worried about specific illnesses than about a more general vulnerability they experience in and through their bodies.

As outlined in the previous section, public health provides one of the frameworks which urban citizens as well as experts use to interpret this experience. From this perspective, urban residents face a broad range of health risks (Harpham and Molyneux 2001) which can be summarized as being a result of high levels of environmental hazards, commoditization, social fragmentation (Moser 1998) and poor governance. Environmental hazards include poor quality of housing and inadequate water supply, sanitation and solid waste disposal. Human excreta, for instance, are extremely dangerous unless safely disposed. Where provisions for water and sanitation are inadequate, the risk of diseases arising from faecal contamination through food, water or hand-to-hand contact is high. People further have to pay for housing, food, water and many other commodities essential for good health. If they face difficulties in generating income, their access to these goods and services is reduced and their health risk increases. In addition to these material risks, citizens are also exposed to problems rooted in the social environment. Greater social heterogeneity in cities may lead to fragmentation and weaken community and intra-household relations of trust and collaboration, especially under conditions of economic hardship. Our findings from Dar es Salaam provide supporting evidence and suggest that these urban health risks combine with many uncertainties and contingencies resulting from global change, poor governance and rapid structural reforms.

In abstract terms, vulnerability can be defined as result of exposure to, and intensity of, health risks in combination with the effectiveness of response options (see Figure 2). This means that, in addition to assessing urban health risks, we need to systematically investigate the options people in a given locality have to resist, overcome or live with these risks.

Ideally, a multilayered analysis of both risks and options with a special focus on the dynamics between these levels should be carried out, especially in urban settings. For the purpose of our study we decided to focus on the household level. We consider households both as a locale and as a normative social arena. Moreover, we see the household as a node between the domestic and the public sphere.

Previous studies of urban households concentrated on "survival strategies" in Middle America (Chant 1991, Gonzàles de la Rocha 1994) and Africa (Hansen 1997, Hoodfar 1997). They documented that urban residents have various options to deal with vulnerability to poverty. We build on their research but ask about response options to urban health risks.

Continuing the systematic approach to the study of everyday health practice introduced in the previous section, we investigate this question empirically, taking the health activities identified by the women as a lead. The range of activities to ensure cleanliness addresses environmental hazards. Most of these activities are prompted by basic public health knowledge which women try to apply. Generating income and food provision are responses to the urban health risk "commoditization". Many study participants emphasized that without financial means, health can hardly be sustained in an urban setting. One of their preoccupations was food insecurity. Child care and health care are activities that help to reduce social fragmentation. As long as people care for weaker members of their families and communities, some basic trust in social relations is sustained.

A basic assumption of our study was that individual women have to interact with others to maintain their own health and that of their families. We introduced the concept of task-centered interactions to investigate these social dynamics, both within the

318

household and in social networks. The term "task" implies that a health activity has to be carried out by somebody. Moreover, this task is assigned to a certain person because she belongs to a social category by virtue of gender, household membership or another principle of social organization. Yet even if a person is responsible for a given task, she interacts with others and does not necessarily carry it out on her own. These social interactions may range from exchanging views and giving advice, granting practical or financial assistance to engaging in negotiations, collaboration or delegation.

We found that for most women (62 percent) the nuclear household constitutes an important social unit in everyday health practice, for instance in the generation of income, in the provision of food and water and in basic hygiene. For even more women (93 percent) the Swahili house community played a central role in the daily management of environmental health, including garbage collection and sanitation. Clear guidelines *(zamu, kuchangia)* regulated who had to contribute what to these activities.

Especially in the late 1990s, informal services were of vital importance in everyday health practice. Since public services such as water supply, garbage collection and human waste disposal were not available, not reliable or not affordable, most people in Ilala Ilala resorted to buying water from street vendors and to paying men to collect the garbage, dig garbage holes or empty cesspits. To a certain extent, we agree with Tripp's (1997) suggestion that people defied the government by changing the rules. The city government banned most of these informal sector services but people did not abide by these regulations. However, we ought to bear in mind that most people did so out of necessity not choice. Whenever we discussed these issues, people asserted they would prefer centralized services at affordable prices. We should not forget that Ilala Ilala is a planned settlement and that government services regularly reached the area.

It should further be noted that some of these "self-help"-solutions aggravate people's health problems. If garbage and human waste is buried in the ground and water pipes are leaky, water-borne diseases are bound to multiply. Many residents of Ilala Ilala are aware of these complex problems, but they see few alternatives. Even after the municipality Ilala took over from the city council and drilled many wells, water safety remained a hotly debated issue, and rightly so in a city of recurrent cholera outbreaks.

Our findings show that even if local options are not always effective, it is crucial to study governance on the household and the community level in particular local realities. Such data are needed to improve good governance from bottom up, for instance with regard to water supply, sanitation and solid waste disposal.

An analysis of women's health options should further pay particular attention to gender as a structuring principle. Similar to other studies, for instance Moore (1994: 55), we found that different, and even contradictory, gender discourses co-exist in this urban society. The majority of women said the household depended on the husband because he was the main breadwinner and authority (N = 74). Smaller groups of women saw the household as dependent on both the parents (N = 14), or themselves (N = 12). Not surprisingly, most women in the last group headed a single-parent household.

Although most women considered their husband as main breadwinner and authority, many men could not live up to this cultural ideal. Indeed, 69 percent of the women had an independent income. Surprisingly, however, nearly all of these women adhered to the dominant gender model. More than half of them (56 percent) spent money on daily food expenses but considered their contribution merely as "help". We assert that this stance should not be interpreted as an indicator of women's low esteem and personal power (see Bruce and Dwyer 1988: 8, Moser 1993: 27). Women rather resisted taking over this additional responsibility and preferred to call their husbands to account. If they were Muslim, they could refer to their right as a wife to depend on the husband (Hoodfar 1997: 270). Women of other ethnic backgrounds and Christian faith also insisted on this right; one of them referred to the Bible to justify her claim. Following (Obbo 1981: 102), we see this as a "non-confrontational method" women employ to improve their situation.

What this means, however, is that most women are not only in charge of reproductive but also of productive tasks. They take care of domestic and personal hygiene, food and water provision, and they pursue income generating activities. Moreover, women have become increasingly involved in day-to-day management of water supply, sanitation and waste removal.

Women and men in Ilala Ilala are exposed to the same urban health risks but women face a heavier burden in mastering them. For this reason we contend that structural constraints of the urban environment have increased gender inequality in everyday health practice. On the other hand, we agree with Tripp (1989: 602) that women are not "simply caught between the dictates of a relentless economic situation and the demands of the husband". Most women in our sample have created a space for negotiations with their husband and children and see the household as a collaborative unit that supports them in their daily struggle for health.

Whether women can mobilize support, and from whom, should be investigated, not assumed. In our study in Dar es Salaam, women first and foremost rely on their husbands. They emphasized how their husbands assisted them in regard to female task fulfillment within the household and in the house community. At the same time, women portrayed themselves as helping their husbands to fulfill their male income generating responsibility. Women also receive much support from children, especially when it comes to cleaning. They sweep the floor, fetch water, wash dishes and help with the laundry. Adolescent girls and boys employed as house helpers are involved in cooking, cleaning and childcare. The few women living in an extended household receive additional help from mothers, mothers-in-law or sisters-in-law, usually in childcare and cooking.

Most women consider giving help to relatives as a moral obligation, irrespective of whether they live in the same or in another household. This help ranges from occasional gifts to substantial support. Relatives took charge of a household when a mother fell ill, or raised the children of parents who could not afford to take care of them. However, a key finding of our study is that this assistance is not given indiscriminately. Even among relatives, support like minding children or helping in setting up an income generating activity is an expression of a special bond, particularly if support is given regularly and/or over a long period, for instance to a handicapped child. While some women insisted on "generalized reciprocity" (Sahlins 1965) as being a kinship obligation (*wajibu kwa familia*), most women in our household sample considered it as help (*msaada*) implying that it was voluntary. We thus suggest that kinship relations – like gender relations – have become subject to reinterpretation.

Moreover, in certain spheres of life the boundaries between relatives, neighbors, friends and work mates have become blurred, for instance where the granting of financial and practical assistance during a sudden crisis or at a life cycle ceremony is concerned. "Balanced reciprocity" (i.e. direct or indirect repayment between two individuals on an equivalent scale) was mainly practiced among fellow tenants and neighbors. If women got along well, they borrowed small sums of money from each other, took turns in watching children while the mother went to the market or helped each other with such items as sugar, onions or tealeaves. This also meant, however, that a woman who was not able to reciprocate faced serious problems in mobilizing support.

What we found especially problematic is that the majority of the women in our sample (65 percent) declared having received financial help only at life cycle ceremonies or in emergencies. Nearly a third (29 percent) reported they did not receive any support outside the household, and a smaller group said they did not give help to others (10 percent). These findings imply that the social "cushion" for many women is rather thin.

Social support networks should not be romanticized. Even if people emphasize the moral obligation to help others, they may not be in a position to give much. On the other hand, some women who say they do not receive any support may not be the ones who need it most. We should, in other words, neither overemphasize nor underestimate the potential of social support networks beyond the household, but investigate them in particular cases instead.

The final and most important question is how the various response options described in this section actually influence vulnerability. Modifying an approach developed by Krüger (1997), we suggest addressing this question by identifying key options. These options can then be further defined by indicators for reduced or increased vulnerability. For our study in Dar es Salaam, we selected the following options: 1) applying public health knowledge to ensure cleanliness, 2) choosing between gender models, 3) mobilizing support within the household, 4) mobilizing support through social networks and groups.

Preliminary as this model is, it enabled us to analyze differentials regarding degrees of vulnerability across households, and to group women along a continuum ranging from least to most vulnerable. It confirmed that vulnerability increases if women are confronted with more urban health risks and have less effective response options. One can also read the model reversely: Women are less vulnerable if they manage to turn some of these options into protective factors.

Our model and the selected indicators clearly need to be further refined and tested in similar study settings. Eventually we should come up with indicators and indexes to measure dimensions of vulnerability to specified urban health risks. The modeling of vulnerability to urban health risks is a pressing need and a rich field for future research.

7.3 Resilience

The third argument of our study is that resilience is a key issue if we want to gain a better understanding of the complex interplay of health and vulnerability on the household level. Up to now not only resilience but also health and vulnerability have hardly been conceptualized in anthropological theory. While health and vulnerability have received increasing attention in neighbouring disciplines like sociology, development studies and geography, resilience has only recently been "discovered" by social scientists working on international development, especially on global environmental change (Kasperson and Kasperson 2001, IHDP Update 2003). In our study, the importance of resilience is a finding, not an idea that guided us throughout data collection; we can therefore only outline what we consider as a new line of inquiry for future research.

Similar to the construct vulnerability, "resilience" has a long history in psychology and psychiatry and has been conceptualized in different ways by different scholars (Weiss 2005). For the purpose of our study we define it as living successfully with urban health risks, i.e. in a socially acceptable and effective way that enhances health and well-being. We suggest taking both local and professional perspectives into account when judging what is "effective" and "enhancing health and well-being".

Such a perspective corresponds with the salutogenic idea of Antonovsky (1979, 1987) which guides our study. An essential salutogenic force is the successful coping with risks and resulting burdens. In addition to coping, Antonovsky's framework identifies a number of generalized resistance resources that refer to bodily, material, psychological, social and cultural aspects. Salutogenic resources develop from the sociocultural context as well as through influences stemming from socialization and individual biography. What he calls "salutogenic resources" refers to our concept of "response options".

This understanding is also similar to contemporary psychological studies on adolescent health and vulnerability, which show that resilience is not a feature or a characteristic some people have and others do not, but an interaction between an individual, his or her family and his or her broader social environment (Blum et al. 2002: 29). The ways in which people interact with their environment can be more or less beneficial to their health, seen from either their own and/or from an expert's point of view.

All these approaches are resource- rather than deficit-oriented. They open a space for the consideration of people as actors, not victims, who shape their lives effectively even under difficult circumstances. As anthropologists we are particularly interested in human agency: We consider individuals as social persons who are capable of reflecting about available knowledge, cultural values and codes of conduct, whether they are enacted or discursive, and to act upon these reflections. We further emphasize practice, i.e. the dialectical relationship between agency and structure. In our study, we made a special effort to make this complex relationship visible. Our data showed that structural conditions forced women to find their own ways of sustaining and restoring health. Each woman had to position herself vis-à-vis structural constraints as well as conventional views and codes of conduct. One woman, for instance, asserted that a person's health is in her own hands. Others formulated critical statements about the applicability of public health to their particular locality. One of them even questioned whether one should talk about "good health" where people lack basic requirements such as financial means and water.

Resilience under conditions of rapid urban change means learning to live with unpredictability and uncertainties that interrupt daily routine. It also means having to deal with diversity. Even when people face comparable urban health risks, they are not equally affected, partly because they make differential use of response options. This means that they act within the context of complex circumstances which sometimes facilitate and sometimes limit what they can do to avoid, overcome or simply live with the consequences of these health risks.

We have used the word "health practice" to suggest that people's health definitions, health explanations and health activities are rooted partly in enacted knowledge, partly in discursive knowledge (see Giddens 1984). Put differently, we see health as a social experience which is both enacted and verbalized. This also implies that resilience is at least partly unfocused, in other words it can mean an ability to improvise, to make ends meet and to balance competing demands and needs. For this reason it is easier to explore and capture local meanings of resilience through participant observation and case studies rather than interviews.

In our research, case studies drew our attention to the fact that women face a series of interrelated dilemmas in health practice. Many response options women have can result in either positive or negative effects on vulnerability. We tried to capture this important finding in the model of socially and culturally relevant resonse options (Figure 3). It not only helped us to systematically investigate the relationship between risks and options but also brings the links between vulnerability and resilience into sharper focus.

As visualized in our model, these dilemmas play on the horizontal level as well as from one level to the next. If we consider, for instance, the first response option "applying public health knowledge", we realize that it may affect women in a positive and a negative way. On the one hand, women can use such knowledge as a resource to turn their home into a healthier place. Seen from this viewpoint, access to health knowledge is a positive option, as long as the messages transmitted are accurate. On the other hand, public health knowledge often turns into a risk when it becomes manifest under the condition we referred to as "delayed medicalization": It may cause emotional distress, especially for those women who have accepted it as a code of values and rules, but cannot put it into practice. Joyce, for example, was highly committed to applying what she had learnt about hygiene: After seeing a commercial for a water filter on TV, however, she was deeply distressed: She could not afford such a filter although it apparently produced drinking water that was safer than boiled water. For several days she seriously debated with herself whether she should continue to spend money on boiling water if it did not really kill all germs. Like many other women, she suffered under the idea that she had to raise her children under such unhygienic conditions. This example illustrates that options may have unexpected and both positive and negative effects.

If we move from horizontal to vertical relations between options, we find that they reinforce each other, again in positive and in negative ways. In many cases that we followed over a period of six months women were caught in a downward spiral; negative outcomes of options had a cumulative effect. These findings suggest that the urban health crisis and subsequent reforms have pushed some women and their households beyond resilience. Their burden grew so heavy that even resourceful women had to give up.

Vulnerability to urban health risks clearly displays a dynamic nature. Options are not only ambiguous and interact synergistically; they also reflect values and codes of conduct which are affected by economic, social and cultural change. If we take women's generalized resistance resources and their response options into account, we see that they live in a complex network of opportunities and constraints. Being resilient and taking an effective and socially acceptable course of action under such circumstances is very difficult indeed. Viewed against this background, "ambivalence coupled with pragmatism" (Lock and Kaufert 1998b: 2) is often the most resilient response.

Nevertheless, our evidence suggests that a better understanding of the complex relationship between vulnerability and resilience may show us a direction towards mitigating urban health risks. Women who are able to combine positive options are obviously in a good position to reduce vulnerability. Such a woman relies partly on her husband and engages him and the children in her daily struggle for health. She earns her own income in a qualified job in the formal sector and runs a sideline activity, for instance a food stall. In order to have reliable assistance in reproductive work within the household, she trains and supervises daughters and house helpers in domestic skills, childcare and health care. With regard to social networks and groups, she carefully maintains a balance between receiving and giving help to relatives, neighbors, work mates and fellow members of voluntary organizations. In our study in Dar es Salaam, few women could live up to this ideal but those who came close were best equipped to sustain the health of their households.

7.4 Conclusions

Our study of household health practice in Bongoland breaks new ground in anthropology by focusing on three closely related concepts – health, vulnerability and resilience – which have been neglected up to now. Grounded in ethnographic data, it develops a systematic approach to the study of health practice. As with all ethnographic data, their internal validity is high but the generalizability is limited to similarly situated communities, i.e. lower-middle class communities in other Tanzanian cities. Comparative research is now needed to test the usefulness of our approach and to refine the framework, models and concepts presented here. Particular attention should be given to the development of indicators that can eventually be measured. Special efforts should be made in the multi-level study of health, vulnerability and resilience. The creation of resilience on individual, social and higher structural levels should become a formidable field for comparative analysis leading to new approaches.

The insights into everyday health practice on the household level provide compelling evidence for the need for a change in policies and interventions. Women's empowerment in terms of income generation and decision making without calling on the husbands to fulfill their share of responsibility towards household health has the opposite effect: It weakens women physically, emotionally and economically and thus has a negative effect on everyday health practice. Women's access to accurate health information from trusted sources should be strengthened. However, Information Education and Communication messages and improvements in water, sanitation and waste removal should be rooted in local realities. Identifying the most appropriate health practice requires intimate knowledge of local conditions, priorities and efforts, as well as of health expertise. Much can be learnt from resilient women but their scope of action is limited. Future approaches should focus on institutional capacities within wards, municipalities and cities that bolster resilience to urban health risks.

Bibliography

Alonzo, A. A. 1993. "Health Behaviour: Issues, Contradictions and Dilemmas." *Social Science and Medicine* 37(8): 1019–1034.

AMMP 1995. *Population Statistics of Surveillance Areas in Dar es Salaam.* Dar es Salaam: Adult Mortality and Morbidity Project (Unpublished Report).

AMMP 1997. *Policy Implications of Adult Morbidity and Mortality. End of Phase 1 Report.* Dar es Salaam: Ministry of Health (Unpublished Report).

Annett, H., Rifkin, S. 1988. *Guidelines for Rapid Appraisal to Assess Community Health Needs. A Focus on Health Improvements for Low-income Urban Areas.* Geneva: WHO (Division of Strengthening of Health Services).

Anonymus 2003. *Government Moves to Privatise Water Supply. East African (Kenya) June 26.* Available at: http://www.hoovnews.hoovers.com/fp/asp (2003, July 15).

Antonovsky, A. 1979. *Health, Stress and Coping: New Perspectives on Mental and Physical Well-being.* San Francisco: Jossey-Bass Publishers.

Antonovsky, A. 1987. *Unraveling the Mistery of Health. How People Manage Stress and Stay Well.* San Francisco: Jossey-Bass Publishers.

Appadurai, A. 1996. *Modernity at Large. Cultural Dimensions of Globalization.* Minneapolis/ London: University of Minnesota Press.

Arcury, T. A., Quant, S. A., and Bell, R. A. 2001. "Staying Healthy: The Salience and Meaning of Health Maintenance Behaviors Among Rural Older Adults in North Carolina." *Social Science and Medicine* 53: 1541–1556.

Ardener, S. 1964. "The Comparative Study of Rotating Credit Associations." *Journal of the Royal Anthropological Institute of Great-Britain and Ireland* 94: 201–230.

Ardener, S., Burman, S., eds. 1995. *Money-Go-Rounds. The Importance of Rotating Saving and Credit Associations for Women.* Oxford, Washington D.C.: Berg Publishers.

Armstrong, D. 1983. *The Political Anatomy of the Body.* Edinburgh: Edinburgh University Press.

Ashton, J. 1991. "Sanitarian Becomes Ecologist: The New Environmental Health." *British Medical Journal* 302: 189–190.

Ashton, J., Seymour, H. 1988. *The New Public Health.* Milton Keynes: Open University Press.

Atkinson, S. 1996. "Applications of Social Research in Urban Health." In *Urban Health Research in Developing Countries. Implications for Policy,* ed. S. Atkinson, J. Songsore, E. Werna. Wallingford: Cab International, pp. 43–64.

Atkinson, S., Songsore, J., Werna, E., eds. 1996. *Urban Health Research in Developing Countries. Implications for Policy.* Wallingford: Cab International.

Baer, H. A., Singer, M., Susser I. 2003. *Medical Anthropology and the World System. A Critical Perspective.* (2nd ed). Westport: Praeger.

Bates, I., Fenton, C., Gruber, J., Lalloo, D., Medina Lara, A., Squire S. B., Theobald, S., Thomson, R., Tolhurst, R. 2004a. "Vulnerability to Malaria, Tuberculosis, and HIV/AIDS Infection and Disease: Part 1: Determinants Operating at Individual and Household Level." *The LANCET Infectious Diseases* 4: 267–277.

Bates, I., Fenton, C., Gruber, J., Lalloo, D., Medina Lara, A., Squire S.B., Theobald, S., Thomson, R., Tolhurst, R. 2004b. "Vulnerability to Malaria, Tuberculosis, and HIV/AIDS Infection and Disease: Part 2: Determinants Operating at Environmental and Institutional Level." *The LANCET Infectious Diseases* 4: 368–375.

Beck, A. 1981. *Medicine, Tradition and Development in Kenya and Tanzania, 1920–1970.* Waltham: Crossroads Press.

Becker, G. 1995. "Medical Anthropology in a Time of Change." *Medical Anthropology Quarterly* 9(1): 3–5.

Beckerleg, S. 1994. "Medical Pluralism and Islam Communities in Kenya." *Medical Anthropology Quarterly* 8(3): 299–313.

Belz-Merk, M. 1995. *Gesundheit ist Alles und alles ist Gesundheit. Die Selbstkonzeptforschung zur Beschreibung und Erklärung subjektiver Vorstellungen von Gesundheit und Gesundheitsverhalten.* Frankfurt a.M.: Peter Lang.

Berman, P., Kendall, C., Bhattacharyya, K. 1994. "The Household Production of Health. Integrating Social Science Perspectives on Micro-Level Health Determinants." *Social Science and Medicine* 38(2): 205–215.

Bibeau, G. 1997. "At Work in the Fields of Public Health. The Abuse of Rationality." *Medical Anthropology Quarterly* 11(2): 246–255.

Blaxter, M. 1990. *Health and Lifestyles.* London: Travistock/Routledge.

Blaxter, M., Paterson, L. 1982. *Mothers and Daughters. A Three-generational Study of Health Attributes and Behaviour.* London: Heinemann.

Blum, R.W., McNeely, C. and Nonnemaker, J. 2002. "Vulnerability, Risk and Protection." *Journal of Adolescent Health* 31: 28–39.

Boesen, J., Havnevik, K.J., Koponen, J., Odgaard, R., eds. 1986. *Tanzania. Crisis and Struggle for Survival.* Uppsala: Scandinavian Institute of African Studies.

Bohle, H.-G. 1994 "Dürrekatastrophen und Hungerkrisen." *Geographische Rundschau,* 7–8: 400–407.

Bohle, H.-G. 2001. "Vulnerability and Criticality: Perspectives for Social Geography." *Update IHDP*: 1–5.

Boot, M. T., Cairncross, S., eds. 1993. *Actions Speak. The Study of Hygiene Behaviour in Water and Sanitation Projects.* The Hague: IRC International Water and Sanitation Centre & London School of Hygiene and Tropical Medicine.

Bott, E. 1957. *Family and Social Networks*. London: Tavistock Publications.

Bourdieu, P. 1977. *Outline of a Theory of Practice*. Cambridge: Cambridge University Press.

Bourdieu, P. 1990. *The Logic of Practice*. Cambridge: Polity Press.

Bruce, J., Dwyer, D. 1988. "Introduction." In *A Home Divided. Women and Income in the Third World*, ed. D. Dwyer, J. Bruce. Stanford: Stanford University Press, pp. 1–19.

Bryceson, D. F. 1990. *Food Insecurity and the Social Division of Labour in Tanzania, 1919–1985*. London: Macmillan.

Brydon, L., Chant, S. 1989. *Women in the Third World. Gender Issues in Rural and Urban Areas*. Aldershot: Edward Elgar.

Bunton, R., MacDonald, G., eds. 1992. *Health Promotion: Disciplines and Diversity*. London: Routledge.

Burke, T. 1996. *Lifebuoy Men, Lux Women. Commodification, Consumption, and Cleanliness in Modern Zimbawe*. London: Leicester University Press.

Calnan, M. 1987. *Health and Illness. The Lay Perspective*. London: Tavistock.

Campbell, J. 1995. "Conceptualizing Gender Relations and the Household in Urban Tanzania." In *Gender, Family and Household in Tanzania*, ed. C. Creighton, C. K. Omari. Aldershot: Avebury, pp. 178–202.

Campbell, J., Mwami, J., Ntukula, M. 1995. "Urban Social Organization. An Exploration of Kinship, Social Networks, Gender Relations and Household and Community in Dar es Salaam." In *Gender, Family and Household in Tanzania*, ed. C. Creighton, C. K. Omari. Aldershot: Avebury, pp. 221–252.

Caudill, W. 1953. "Applied Anthropology in Medicine." In *Anthropology Today. An Encyclopedic Inventory*, ed. A. L. Kroeber. Chicago: The University of Chicago Press, pp. 771–806.

Chaligha A. E. 2002. *Local Government in Tanzania*. Available at: http://tanzania.fes-international.de/Activities/Docs/LocalGovernment.html (2004, May 9).

Chambers, R. 1989. "Editorial Introduction. Vulnerability, Coping and Policy." *How the Poor Cope. IDS-Bulletin* 20(2): 1–7.

Chant, S. 1989. "Gender and the Urban Household." In *Women in the Third World. Gender Issues in Rural and Urban Areas*, ed. L. Brydon, S. Chant. New Brunswick: Rutgers University Press, pp. 134–160.

Chant, S. 1991. *Women and Survival in Mexican Cities. Perspectives on Gender, Labour Markets and Low-income Households*. Manchester: Manchester University Press.

Chant, S. 1997. *Women-headed Households. Diversity and Dynamics in the Developing World*. London: Macmillan.

Chavunduka, G. L. 1978. *Traditional Healers and the Shona Patient*. Salisbury: Mambo Press.

Chrisman, N. J. 1977. "The Health Seeking Process. An Approach to the Natural History of Illness." *Culture, Medicine and Psychiatry* 1: 351–377.

Cohn, R. C. 1997. *Von der Psychoanalyse zur themenzentrierten Interaktion. Von der Behandlung einzelner zu einer Pädagogik für alle (13th ed.).* Stuttgart: Klett-Cotta.

Corbett, J. 1989. "Poverty and Sickness. The High Costs of Ill-health." *How the Poor Cope. IDS-Bulletin* 20(2): 58–62.

Coreil, J., Mull, J. B., eds. 1990. *Anthropology and Primary Health Care.* Boulder: Westview Press.

Crawford, R. 1977. "You Are Dangerous to Your Health. The Ideology of Victim Blaming." *International Journal of Health Services* 7(3): 663–680.

Crawford, R. 1980. "Healthism and the Medicalisation of Everyday Life." *International Journal of Health Services* 10(3): 365–388.

Crawford, R. 1987. "Cultural Influences on Prevention and the Emergence of a New Health Consciousness." In *Taking Care. Understanding and Encouraging Self-protective Behaviour,* ed. N. D. Weinstein. Cambridge: Cambridge University Press, pp. 95–113.

Creighton, C., Omari, C. K. 1995. *Gender, Family and Household in Tanzania.* Aldershot: Avebury.

Csordas, T. J. 1990. "Embodiment as a Paradigm for Anthropology." *Ethos* 18: 5–47.

Curtis, V. 1998. *The Dangers of Dirt. Household Hygiene and Health.* Ph. D. thesis, Landbouwuniversiteit Wageningen. Wageningen: Grafisch Service Centrum.

Darch, C. 1996. *Tanzania* (World Bibliographical Series, 54). Oxford: Clio Press.

Das, V. 1990. "What Do We Mean by Health?" In *What We Know About Health Transition. The Cultural, Social and Behavioural Determinants of Health,* ed. J. Caldwell, S. Findley, P. Caldwell, G. Santow, W. Cosford, J. Braid and D. Broers-Freeman. Canberra: Health Transition Centre, the Australian National University, pp. 27–46.

DAWASA 1999–2003. *Introduction.* Available at: http://www.dawasa.org (2004, April 28).

Delor, F., Hubert, M. 2000. "Revisiting the Concept of Vulnerability." *Social Science and Medicine* 50: 1557–1570.

D'Houtard, A., Field, M. G. 1984. "The Image of Health. Variations in Perceptions by Social Class in a French Population." *Sociology of Health and Illness* 6: 30–60.

Douglas, M. 1975. *Implicit Meanings.* London, New York: Routledge and Regan Publishers.

Douglas, M. 1992. *Risk and Blame. Essays in Cultural Theory.* London, New York: Routledge.

Douglas, M., Wildavsky, A. 1982. *Risk and Culture.* Berkeley: California University Press.

Downie, R.S., Tannahill, C., Tannahill, A. 1996. *Health Promotion. Models and Values*. Oxford: Oxford University Press.

DUHP 2004. *Dar es Salaam Urban Health Project. A Project for Improving Health Care Delivery and health promotion in urban Tanzania*. Dar es Salaam: Dar es Salaam City Council, City Medical Office of Health, Basel: Swiss Tropical Institute, Swiss Centre for International Health (CD ROM).

Duque, J., Pastrana, E. 1973. *Las estrategias de supervivencia económica de las unidades familiares del sector popular urbano: una investigación exploratoria*. Santiago de Chile: Facultad Latino-americana de Ciencias Sociales (FLASCO).

Dwyer, D., Bruce, J., eds. 1988. *A Home Divided. Women and Income in the Third World*. Stanford: Stanford University Press.

Evans, T. 1989. "The Impact of Permanent Disability on Rural Households. River Blindness in Guinea." *How the Poor Cope. IDS-Bulletin* 20(2): 41–48.

Fabrega, H. 1972. "Medical Anthropology." In *Biennial Review of Anthropology*, ed. B.J. Siegel. Stanford: Stanford University Press, pp. 167–229.

Faltermaier, T. 1994. *Gesundheitsbewusstsein und Gesundheitshandeln*. Weinheim: Beltz.

Faltermaier, T., Kühnlein, I., Burda-Viering, M. 1998. *Gesundheit im Alltag. Laienkompetenz in Gesundheitshandeln und Gesundheitsförderung*. Weinheim, München: Juventa.

Fapohunda, E. 1988. "The Non-pooling Household. A Challenge to Theory." In *A Home Divided. Women and Income in the Third World*, ed. D. Dwyer and J. Bruce. Stanford: Stanford University Press, pp. 143–154.

Featherstone, M. 2002. *Global Culture. Nationalism, Globalization and Modernity*. London: Sage.

Feierman, S., Janzen, J.M., eds. 1992. *The Social Basis of Health and Healing in Africa*. Berkeley, Los Angeles, Oxford: University of California Press.

Fidelis, M. 1994. *The Plight of Housegirls in Tanzania. A Case Study of Dar es Salaam Region*. BA dissertation, Dar es Salaam: Department of Sociology, University of Dar es Salaam.

Fiedler, I. 1983. *Wandel in der Mädchenerziehung in Tanzania*. Saarbrücken: Breitenbach Publishers.

Finch, J., Mason, J. 1993. *Negotiating Family Responsibilities*. London, New York: Tavistock/Routledge.

Fjeldstad, O.-H. 2004. *To Pay or not to Pay? Citizen's views on taxation in local authorities in Tanzania*. Paper presented at the REPOAs 9th Annual Research Workshop, Dar es Salaam, 25–26 March. Available at: http://www.cmi.no/research (2004, May 5).

Fjeldstad, O.-H., Chaligha, A. and Braathen, E. 2003. *Formative Research Project on Local Government Reform in Tanzania*. Project Brief, No. 1. Available at: http://www.cmi.no/publications (2004, July 31).

Flick, U., ed. 1991. *Alltagswissen über Gesundheit und Krankheit. Subjektive Theorien und soziale Repräsentationen.* Heidelberg: Roland Asanger.

Flick, U., ed. 1998. *Wann fühlen wir uns gesund? Subjektive Vorstellungen von Gesundheit und Krankheit.* Weinheim, München: Juventa.

Foster, G. 1994. *Hippocrates' Latin American Legacy. Humoral Medicine in the New World.* Langhorne: Gordon and Breach.

Foucault, M. 1961. *Folie et déraison. Histoire de la folie à l'âge classique.* Paris: Plon.

Foucault, M. 1963. *Naissance de la clinique. Une archéologie du regard médical.* Paris: Presses Universitaires de France.

Foucault, M. 1984. *Histoire de la Sexualité. L'usage des plaisirs.* Paris: Editions Gallimard.

Fuglesang, M. 1997. "Lessons for Life. Past and Present Modes of Sexuality Education in Tanzania Society." *Social Science and Medicine* 44(8): 1245–1254.

Geertz, C. 1962. "The Rotating Credit Association. A 'Middle Ring' in Development." *Economic Development and Cultural Change* 10: 241–263.

Giddens, A. 1979. *Central Problems in Social Theory. Action, Structure and Contradiction in Social Analysis.* Berkeley, Los Angeles: University of California Press.

Giddens, A. 1984. *The Constitution of Society. Outline of the Theory of Structuration.* Cambridge: Polity Press.

Gilbert, A., Gugler, J. 1994. *Cities, Poverty and Development. Urbanization in the Third World* (2nd ed.). Oxford: Oxford University Press.

Gmelch, G., Zenner, W.P. 1996. *Urban Life. Readings in Urban Anthropology* (3rd ed.). Prospect Heights: Waveland Press.

González de la Rocha, M. 1994. *The Resources of Poverty. Women and Survival in a Mexican City.* Oxford: Blackwell.

Good, B. J. 1994. *Medicine, Rationality, and Experience. An Anthropological Perspective.* Cambridge: Cambridge University Press.

GTZ (Deutsche Gesellschaft für Technische Zusammenarbeit), 2001. *Urban Health: Particularities, Challenges, Experiences and Lessons Learnt: A Literature Review.* Eschborn: GTZ.

Guène, O., Touré, C.S., Maystre, L.Y. 1999. *Promotion de l'hygiène du milieu. Une stratégie participative, collection gérer l'environnement 17.* Lausanne: Presses polytechniques et universitaires romandes.

Gugler, J., ed. 1988. *The Urbanization of the Third World.* Oxford: Oxford University Press.

Guyer, J. 1997. "Households." In *The Dictionary of Anthropology,* ed. T. Barfield. Oxford: Blackwell Publishers, pp. 245–246.

Guyer, J. I. 1981. "Household and Community in African Studies." *African Studies Review* 24(2/3): 87–137.

Guyer, J., Peters, P. 1987. "Introduction." *Development and Change* 18: 197–214.

Hall, B. L. 1978. *Mtu ni Afya. Tanzania's Health Campaign.* Washington: Clearinghouse.

Hannerz, U. 1992. *Cultural Complexity. Studies in the Social Organization of Meaning*. New York: Columbia Press.

Hansen, K. T. 1997. *Keeping House in Lusaka*. New York: Columbia University Press.

Harcourt, W., ed. 1997. *Power, Reproduction and Gender. The Intergenerational Transfer of Knowledge*. London, New Jersey: Zed Books.

Harpham, T. 1996. "Urban Health Research in Developing Countries. Reflections on the Last Decade." In *Urban Health Research in Developing Countries. Implications for Policy*, ed. S. Atkinson, J. Songsore, E. Werna. Wallingford: Cab International, pp. 1–9.

Harpham, T., Lusty, T., Vaughan, P. 1988. *In the Shadow of the City. Community Health and the Urban Poor*. Oxford: Oxford University Press.

Harpham, T., Molyneux, C. 2001. "Urban Health in Developing Countries: A Review." *Progress in Development Studies* 1(2): 113–137.

Harpham, T., Tanner, M., eds. 1995. *Urban Health in Developing Countries. Progress and Prospects*. London: Earthscan.

Harts-Broekhuis, A. 1997. "How to Sustain a Living? Urban Households and Poverty in the Sahelian Town of Mopti." *Africa* 67(1): 106–129.

Heggenhoughen, H. K. 1986. "Health Services. Official and Inofficial." In *Tanzania. Crisis and Struggle for Survival*, ed. J. Boesen, K. J. Havnevik, J. Koponen, R. Odgaard. Uppsala: Scandinavian Institute of African Studies, pp. 309–317.

Heggenhoughen, K., Vaughan, P., Muhondwa, E. P. Y., Rutabanzibwa-Ngaiza, J. 1987. *Community Health Workers. The Tanzanian Experience*. Oxford: Oxford University Press.

Heinrich, T. 1987. *Technologietransfer in der Stadtplanung. Masterplanung in Dar es Salaam, Tansania durch internationale Consultings*. Darmstadt: Verlag für Wissenschaftliche Publikationen.

Helman, C. 2000. *Culture, Health and Illness*. 4th ed. Oxford: Butterworth and Heinemann.

Herzlich, C. 1969. *Santé et maladie. Analyse d'une représentation sociale*. Paris: Ecole des Hautes Études en Science Sociale (Engl. Transl. *Health and Illness*. London: Academic Press 1973).

Herzlich, C. 1998. „Soziale Repräsentation von Gesundheit und Krankheit und ihre Dynamik im sozialen Feld." In *Wann fühlen wir uns gesund? Subjektive Vorstellungen von Gesundheit und Krankheit*, ed. U. Flick. Weinheim, München: Juventa, pp. 171–180.

Heuveline, P., Guillot, M. and Gwatkin, D. R. 2002. "The Uneven Tides of the Health Transition." *Social Science and Medicine*. 55(2): 313–322.

Hoodfar, H. 1988. "Household Budgeting and Financial Management in a Lower-income Cairo Neighbourhood." In *A Home Divided. Women and Income in the Third World*, ed. D. Dwyer, J. Bruce. Stanford CA: Stanford University Press, pp. 120–142.

337

Hoodfar, H. 1997. *Between Marriage and the Market. Intimate Politics and Survival in Cairo.* Berkeley, Los Angeles, London: University of California Press.

IHDP Update. 2003. *Newsletter of the International Human Dimensions Programme on Global Environmental Change* 02. Available at: http://www.ihdp.org (2004, July 9).

Janzen, J. M. 1978. *The Quest for Therapy in Lower Zaire.* Berkeley, London: University of California Press.

Janzen, J. M. 1997. "Healing." In *Encyclopedia of Africa South of the Sahara,* vol.2, ed. J. Middleton. New York: Simon & Schuster, Macmillan, pp. 274–283.

Johnson, B. B., Covello, V. T., eds. 1987. *The Social and Cultural Construction of Risk. Essays on Risk Selection and Perception.* Dordrecht, Boston, Lancaster, Tokyo: D. Reidel Publishing Company.

Kaitilla, S. 1990. "Low Cost Urban Renewal in Tanzania. Community Participation in Dar-Es-Salaam." *Cities* (August): 211–223.

Kasl, S. V., Cobb, S. 1966. "Health Behaviour, Illness Behaviour and Sick Role Behaviour." *Archives of Environmental Health* 12: 246–266.

Kasperson, J. X., Kasperson R. E. 2001. *International Workshop on Vulnerability and Global Environmental Change.* (Unpubl. Report) Stockholm Environment Institute.

Kindig, D., Stoddart, G. 2003. "What is Population Health?" *American Journal of Public Health,* 93(3): 380–383.

King, A. 1990. *Global Cities.* London: Routledge.

Kleinman, A. 1980. *Patients and Healers in the Context of Culture. An Exploration of the Borderland between Anthropology, Medicine and Psychiatry.* Berkeley: University of California Press.

Kleinman, A., Veena, D., Lock, M., eds. (1997) *Social Suffering.* Berkeley: University of California Press.

Koda, B. O., Omari, C. K. 1991. "Crisis in the Household Economy. Women's Strategies in Dar es Salaam." In *Alternative Strategies for Africa,* vol. 2., ed. M. Suliman. London: Institute for African Alternatives, pp. 117–131.

Koda, B. O. 1995. "The Economic Organization of the Household in Contemporary Tanzania." In *Gender, Family and Household in Tanzania,* ed. C. Creighton, C. K. Omari. Aldershot: Avebury, pp. 139–155.

Köhler, M. 1988. "Die Geschichte Ostafrikas seit der Zeitwende." In *Richtig Reisen. Ostafrika: Kenya – Tanzania – Uganda – Rwanda – Burundi,* ed. M. Köhler. Köln: DuMont, pp. 89–145.

Koning, K. de, Martin, M., eds. 1996. *Participatory Research in Health. Issues and Experiences.* London, New Jersey: Zed Books Ltd., Johannesburg: NPPHCN.

Koning, K. de. 1994. *Proceedings of the International Symposium on Participatory Research in Health Promotion.* Liverpool: Liverpool School of Tropical Medicine.

Koponen, J. 1994. *Development for Exploitation. German Colonial Policies in Mainland Tanzania, 1884–1914.* (Studien zur Afrikanischen Geschichte, 10). Münster: Lit.

Krüger, F. D. 1997. *Urbanisierung und Verwundbarkeit in Botswana. Existenzsicherung und Anfälligkeit städtischer Bevölkerungsgruppen in Gaborone.* Pfaffenweiler: Centaurus.

Krüger, F., Macamo, E. 2003. "Existenzsicherung unter Risikobedingungen. Sozialwissenschaftliche Analyseansätze zum Umgang mit Krisen, Konflikten und Katastrophen." *Geographica Helvetica* 58(1): 47–55.

Kulaba, S. 1989. "Local Government and the Management of Urban Services in Tanzania." In *African Cities in Crisis. Managing Rapid Urban Growth,* ed. R. E. Stren, R. R. White. Boulder (San Francisco), London: Westview Press, pp. 203–245.

Labisch, A. 1992. *Homo Hygienicus. Gesundheit und Medizin in der Neuzeit.* Frankfurt, New York: Campus Verlag.

Lamphere, L., Ragoné, H., Zavella, P. 1997. *Situated Lives. Gender and Culture in Everyday Life.* New York, London: Routledge.

Landberg, P. 1986. "Widows and Divorced Women in Swahili Society." In *Widows in African Societies. Choices and Constraints,* ed. B. Potash. Stanford: Stanford University Press, pp. 107–129.

Larsen, K. 1998. "Morality and the Rejection of Spirits. A Zanzibari Case." *Social Anthropology* 6(1): 61–75.

Legum, C., Mmari, G., eds. 1995. *Mwalimu. The Influence of Nyerere.* London: Britain-Tanzania Society.

Leslie, C., ed. 1976. *Asian Medical Systems. A Comparative Study.* Berkeley, Los Angeles, London: University of California Press.

Leslie, C., Young, A., eds. 1992. *Paths to Asian Medical Knowledge.* Berkeley, Los Angeles, London: University of California Press.

Leslie, J. A. K. 1963. *A Survey of Dar es Salaam.* London, New York, Nairobi: Oxford University Press.

Lewis, O. 1959. *Five Families: Mexican Case Studies in the Culture of Poverty.* New York: Basic Books.

Lewis, O. 1961. *The Children of Sánchez.* Middlesex: Penguin Books.

Lloyd, P. 1979. *Slums of Hope? Shanty Towns in the Third World.* Harmondsworth: Penguin.

Lock, M., Kaufert, P. A. 1998a. *Pragmatic Women and Body Politics.* Cambridge: Cambridge University Press.

Lock, M., Kaufert, P. A. 1998b. "Introduction." In *Pragmatic Women and Body Politics,* ed. M. Lock and P. A. Kaufert. Cambridge: Cambridge University Press, pp. 1–27.

Lomnitz, L. A. 1977. *Neworks and Marginality. Life in a Mexican Shanty Town.* New York: Academic.

Lomnitz, L. A. 1988. "Informal Exchange Networks in Formal Systems. A Theoretical Model." *American Anthropologist* 90: 42–55.

Lugalla, J. 1995. *Crisis, Urbanization and Urban Poverty in Tanzania. A Study of Urban Poverty and Survival Politics.* Lanham, New York, London: University Press of America.

Lupton, D. 1999. *Risk.* London, New York: Routledge.

Maliyamkono, T. L., Bagachwa, M. S. D. 1990. *The Second Economy in Tanzania.* London: Currey.

Manderson, L. 1996. *Sickness and the State. Health and Illness in Colonial Malaya 1870–1940.* Cambridge: Cambridge University Press.

Manderson, L., Aaby, P. 1992. "An Epidemic in the Field? Rapid Assessment Procedures and Health Research." *Social Science and Medicine* 35(7): 839–850.

Mascarenhas, A. 1967. "The Impact of Nationhood on Dar es Salaam." *East African Geographical Review* 5: 39–46.

Massé, R. 1995. *Culture et santé publique.* Montréal, Paris, Casablanca: Gaëtan Morin.

Mazrui, A. M., Shariff, I. N. 1994. *The Swahili. Idiom and Identity of an African People.* Trenton NJ: Africa World Press.

McCauley, A. P., West, S., Lynch, M. 1992. "Household Decisions Among the Gogo People of Tanzania. Determining the Roles of Men, Women and the Community in Implementing a Trachoma Prevention Program." *Social Science and Medicine* 34(6): 817–824.

McDowell, I., Newell, C. 1996. *Measuring Health. A Guide to Rating Scales and Questionnaires (2nd ed.).* Oxford, New York: Oxford University Press.

McElroy, A. 1996. "Medical Anthropology." In *Encyclopedia of Cultural Anthropology,* ed. D. Levinson, M. Ember. New York: Henry Holt, pp. 759–763.

McGranahan, G., Jacobi, P., Songsore, J., Surjadi, C., Kjellen, M. 2001. *The Citizens at Risk: From Urban Sanitation to Sustainable Cities.* London: Earthscan.

McGranahan, G., Songsore, J. 1996. "Wealth, Health, and the Urban Household. Weighing Environmental Burdens in Accra, Jakarta, and Sao Paulo." In *Urban Health Research in Developing Countries. Implications for Policy,* ed. S. Atkinson, J. Songsore, E. Werna. Wallingford: Cab International, pp. 135–159.

McGranahan, G., Songsore, J., Kjellén, M. 1996. "Sustainability, Poverty and Urban Environmental Transitions." In *Sustainability, the Environment and Urbanization,* ed. C. Pugh. London: Earthscan, pp. 103–133.

Middleton, J. 1992. *The World of the Swahili. An African Mercantile Civilization.* New Haven: Yale University Press.

Milbert, I., Peat, V. 1999. *What Future for Urban Cooperation? Assessment of Post Habitat II Strategies.* Bern: Swiss Agency for Development and Cooperation (SDC).

Mitchell, J. C., ed. 1969. *Social Networks in Urban Situations.* Manchester: Manchester University Press.

Mitlin, D., Thompson, J. 1995. "Participatory Approaches in Urban Areas. Strengthening Civil Society or Reinforcing the Status Quo?" *Environment and Urbanization* 7(1): 231–250.

Moore, H. 1988. *Feminism and Anthropology.* Cambridge: Polity Press.

Morduch, J. 1999. "Between the State and the Market: Can Informal Insurance Patch the Safety Net?" *The World Bank Research Observer* 14(2): 187–207.

Moser, C. 1993. *Gender Planning and Development: Theory, Practice and Training.* London, New York: Routledge.

Moser, C. 1998. "The Asset Vulnerability Framework: Reassessing Urban Poverty Reduction Strategies." *World Development* 26(1): 1–19.

Mpangile, G.S., Leshabari, T., Kihwele, D.J. 1993. "Factors Associated with Induced Abortion in Public Hospitals in Dar es Salaam." *Reproductive Health Matters* 2: 21–31.

Mwami, J.A.L. 1991. *Coping in a Town. The Case of Low-income Households in Mvuleni (Manzese), Dar es Salaam.* M.A. thesis sociology, University of Dar es Salaam (Unpublished).

N'Diaye, M. 1999. "Recherche populaire." In *Environnement urbain. Recherche et action dans les pays en développement,* ed. J.-C. Bolay, P. Odermatt, Y. Pedrazzini, M. Tanner. Basel, Boston, Berlin: Birkhäuser Verlag, pp. 23–28.

Newell K., ed. 1975. *Health by the People.* Geneva: World Health Organization.

Ngubane, H. 1977. *Body and Mind in Zulu Medicine. An Ethnography of Health and Disease in Nyuswa-Zulu Thought and Practice.* London: Academic Press.

Nichter, M., Lock, M. eds. 2002. *New Horizons in Medical Anthropology. Essays in Honour of Charles Leslie.* London: Routledge.

Nichter, M., Nichter, M. 1996. *Anthropology and International Health. Asian Case Studies.* Amsterdam: OPA.

Nyerere, J.K. 1969. "Ujamaa – the Basis of African Socialism." In *Self-reliant Tanzania,* ed. K.E. Svendsen, M. Teisen. Dar es Salaam: Tanzania Publishing House, pp. 158–167.

Obbo, C. 1981. *African Women. Their Struggle for Economic Independence.* London: Zed Press.

Obrist van Eeuwijk, B. 1996. "The Discovery of Qualitative Approaches in Health Research." *Tsantsa* 1: 71–75.

Obrist van Eeuwijk, B. 1998. "Gesundheit, Umwelt und städtische Entwicklung in Dar es Salaam," *Medicus Mundi* 71: 23–25.

Obrist van Eeuwijk, B. 1999a. "'Blyb Gsund' in Dar es Salaam, Tansania." *UNI NOVA* 85: 42–45.

Obrist van Eeuwijk, B. 1999b. Editorial "Urban Health and Household Decision-making." *Tropical Medicine and International Health* 4.2: 77–78.

Obrist van Eeuwijk, B. 2002a. "Gesundheit in Städten der Dritten Welt. Ein Graduiertenprogramm des Schweizerischen Tropeninstitut und des Ethnologischen Seminars der Universität Basel." In *Schweizerische Akademie* der Geistes- und Sozialwissenschaften, Forschungspartnerschaft mit Entwicklungsländern. Eine Herausforderung für die Geistes- und Sozialwissenschaften, Bern: Schweizerische Akademie der Geistes- und Sozialwissenschaften, pp. 49–54.

Obrist van Eeuwijk, B. 2002b. "Gesundheitsverständnis im Wandel. Perspektiven aus Afrika." UNI PRESS 112: 45–47.

Obrist van Eeuwijk, B. 2002c. "Ohne Sauberkeit keine Gesundheit. Hygiene im Alltag von Dar es Salaam, Tansania." Tsantsa 7: 66–76.

Obrist van Eeuwijk, B., Mdungi, Z. N. 1995. "'Upatu kwa Afya.' Supporting Women's Solidarity Initiatives in Low-income Urban Areas of Dar es Salaam, Tanzania." In Überleben im afrikanischen Alltag – L'Afrique part tous les matins, ed. B. Sottas, L. Roost Vischer. Bern: Peter Lang, pp. 143–158.

Obrist van Eeuwijk, B., Mlangwa, S. 1997. "Competing Ideologies: Adolescence, Knowledge and Silences in Dar es Salaam." In Power, Reproduction and Gender. The Intergenerational Transfer of Knowledge, ed. W. Harcourt. London, New Jersey: Zed Books.

Obrist van Eeuwijk, B., Minja, H. 1997. "Reconsidering the Concept of Household Headship. Reflections on Women's Notions and Practices of Headship in Dar es Salaam, Tanzania." In Werkschau Afrikastudien – Le forum suisse des africanistes, ed. B. Sottas, T. Hammer, L. Roost Vischer, A. Mayor. Hamburg: Lit Verlag, pp. 209–222.

Obrist van Eeuwijk, B., Tanner, M. 2002. "Building Research Networks and Partnerships." Urban Health and Development Bulletin 5.3&4: 5–10.

Obrist, B. 2003. "Urban Health in Daily Practice. Livelihood, Vulnerability and Resilience in Dar es Salaam, Tanzania." Anthropology and Medicine 10.3: 275–290.

Obrist, B. 2004a. "Medicalization and Morality in a Weak State: Health, Hygiene and Water in Dar es Salaam." Anthropology and Medicine Volume 11/01, 43–57.

Obrist, B. (n. d.) Daily Governance of Environmental Health. Gender Perspectives from Dar es Salaam. (In press)

Obrist, B., Eeuwijk P. van. eds. 2003. "Afflictions of City Life. Accounts from Africa and Asia." Anthropology and Medicine (Special Issue) 10.3.

Obrist, B., Tanner M., Harpham, T. 2003b. "Engaging Anthropology in Urban Health Research: Issues and Prospects." Anthropology and Medicine 10.3: 361–371.

Obrist, B., Weiss M. G., Eeuwijk, P. van. 2003a. "Health Anthropology and Urban Health Research." Anthropology and Medicine 10.3: 267–274.

Odermatt, P., Cissé, G., Tanner, M. 1999. "Quelle approche pour quel type de recherche?" In Environnement urbain. Recherche et action dans les pays en développement, ed. J.-C. Bolay, P. Odermatt, Y. Pedrazzini, M. Tanner. Basel, Boston, Berlin: Birkhäuser Verlag, pp. 29–37.

Omari, C.K. 1995b. "The Management of Tribal and Religious Diversity." In *Mwalimu. The Influence of Nyerere*, ed. C. Legum, G. Mmari. London: James Currey, pp. 23–31.

Omari, C.K. 1995a. "Decision-making and the Household: Case Studies from Tanzania." In *Gender, Family and Household in Tanzania*, ed. C. Creighton, C.K. Omari. Aldershot: Avebury, pp. 203–220.

Omran, A.R. 1971. "The Epidemiological Transition: A Theory of the Epidemiology of Population Change." *Milbank Memorial Fund Quarterly* 49: 509–538.

Oppong, C. 1981. *Middle Class African Marriage. A Family Study of Ghanaian Senior Civil Servants*. London: Allen & Unwin.

Ortner, S.B. 1984. "Theory in Anthropology Since the Sixties." *Comparative Studies in Society and History* 26: 126–166.

Ortner, S., Whitehead, H. 1981. *Sexual Meanings: The Cultural Construction of Gender and Sexuality*. Cambridge: Cambridge University Press.

Papanek, H., Schwede, L. 1988. "Women Are Good with Money. Earning and Managing in an Indonesian City." In *A Home Divided. Women and Income in the Third World*, ed. D. Dwyer, J. Bruce. Standford: Stanford University Press, pp. 71–98.

Petersen, A., Lupton, D. 1996. *The New Public Health. Health and Self in the Age of Risk*. London: Sage Publications.

Phillips D.R. 1993. "Urbanization and Human Health." *Parasitology* 106: 93–107.

Pill, R., Stott, N. 1982. "Concepts of Illness Causation and Responsibility. Some Preliminary Data from a Sample of Working Class Mothers." *Social Science and Medicine* 16(1): 43–52.

Pill, R., Stott, N. 1985a. "Choice or Chance. Further Evidence on Ideas of Illness and Responsibility for Health." *Social Science and Medicine* 20(10): 981–991.

Pill, R., Stott, N. 1985b. "Preventive Procedures and Practices Among Working Class Women. New Data and Fresh Insights." *Social Science and Medicine* 21(9): 975–983.

Pill, R., Stott, N. 1987. "Development of a Measure of Potential Health Behaviour: A Salience of Lifestyle Index." *Social Science and Medicine* 24(2): 125–134.

Polgar, S. 1962. "Health and Human Behavior. Areas of Interest Common to the Social and Medical Sciences." *Current Anthropology* 3: 159–205.

Pollard, T.M., Hyatt, S.B., eds. 1999. *Sex, Gender and Health*. Cambridge: Cambridge University Press.

Population and Housing Census 2002. *General Report*. Available at: http://www.tanzania.go.tz/census.dsm.htm. (2004, July 31).

Press, I. 1971. "The Urban Curandero." *American Anthropologist* 73: 741–756.

Pryer, J. 1989. "When Breadwinners Fall Ill. Preliminary Findings from a Case Study in Bangladesh." *How the Poor Cope. IDS-Bulletin* 20(2): 49–57.

Pugh, C. 1996. "Sustainability and Sustainable Cities." In *Sustainability, the Environment and Urbanization*, ed. C. Pugh. London: Earthscan, pp. 135–177.

Ritenbaugh, C. 1982. "Obesity as Culture-bound Syndrome." *Culture, Medicine and Psychiatry* 6: 347–361.

Robinson, D., ed. 1985. *Epidemiology and the Community Control of Disease in Warm Climate Countries* (2nd ed.). Edinburgh, London, Melbourne, New York: Churchill Livingstone.

Roost, Vischer, L. 1997. *Mütter zwischen Herd und Markt. Das Verhältnis von Mutterschaft, sozialer Elternschaft und Frauenarbeit bei den Moose (Mossi) in Ouagadougou/Burkina Faso* (Basler Beiträge zur Ethnologie 38). Basel: Ethnologisches Seminar der Universität und Museum der Kulturen Basel.

Rothman, K. J., Greenland, S., eds. 1998. *Modern Epidemiology* (2nd ed.) Philadelphia: Lippincott-Raven.

Sahlins, M. D. 1965. "On the Sociology of Primitive Exchange." In *The Relevance of Models for Social Anthropology*, ed. M. Banton (ASA Monographs, No. 1). London: Academic Press, pp. 139–236.

Salem, G., Jeannée, E., eds. 1989. *Urbanisation et santé dans le tiers monde. Transition épidémiologique, changement social et soins de santé primaires*. Paris: Editions de l'ORSTOM.

Saltonstall, R. 1993. "Healthy Bodies, Social Bodies: Men's and Women's Concepts and Practice of Health in Everyday Life." *Social Science and Medicine* 36(1): 1–14.

Sanjek, R. 1990. "Urban Anthropology in the 1980s. A World View." *Annual Review of Anthropology* 19: 151–186.

Satterthwaite, D. 1993. "The Impact on Health of Urban Environments." *Environment and Urbanization* 5.2: 87–111.

Scheper-Hughes, N. 1992. *Death Without Weeping. The Violence of Everyday Life in Brazil*. Berkeley, Los Angeles, Oxford: University of California Press.

Scheper-Hughes, N., Lock, M. 1987. "The Mindful Body. A Prolegomenon to Future Work in Medical Anthropology." *Medical Anthropology Quarterly* 1.1: 6–41.

Schipperges, H. 1987. *Der Garten der Gesundheit. Medizin im Mittelalter*. München, Zürich: Artemis Velag.

Schmink, M. 1984. "Household Economic Strategies. Review and Research Agenda." *Latin American Research Review* 19(3): 87–101.

Schulz-Burgdorf, U. 1994. *Aspekte der Swahili-Volksmedizin im Lamu-Archipel Kenyas*. Münster: Lit Verlag.

Schweizer, T., White, D. R., eds. 1998. *Kinship, Networks and Exchange* (Structural Analysis in the Social Sciences 12). Cambridge: Cambridge University Press.

Scotch, N. A. 1963. "Medical Anthropology." In *Biennial Review of Anthropology*, ed. B. J. Siegel. Stanford: Stanford University Press, pp. 30–68.

Scott, J.C. 1985. *Weapons of the Weak. Everyday Forms of Peasant Resistance.* New Haven: Yale University Press.

Selby, H.A., Murphy, A.D., Lorenzen, S. 1990. *The Mexican Urban Household. Organizing Self-Defence.* Austin: University of Texas Press.

Sen, A. K. 1990. "Gender and Cooperative Conflicts." In *Persistent Inequalities. Women and World Development,* ed. I. Tinker. New York: Oxford University Press, pp. 123–149.

Simon, D. 1992. *Cities, Capital and Development. African Cities in the World Economy.* London: Belhaven Press.

Singer, M., Baer, H. 1995. *Critical Medical Anthropology.* Amityville: Baywood.

Songsore, J., McGranahan, G. 1998. "The Political Economy of Household Environmental Management. Gender, Environment and Epidemiology in the Greater Accra Metropolitan Area." *World Development* 26(3): 395–412.

Songsore, J., McGranahan, G. 1993. "Environment, Wealth and Health. Towards an Analysis of Intra-Urban Differentials Within the Greater Accra Metropolitan Area, Ghana." *Environment and Urbanization* 5(2): 10–34.

Songsore, J., Nabila, J.S., Amuzu, A.T., Tutu, K.A., Yangyuoru, Y., McGranahan, G., Kjellén, M. 1998. *Proxy Indicators for Rapid Assessment of Environmental Health Status of Residential Areas. The Case of the Greater Accra Metropolitan Area (GAMA), Ghana* (Urban Environment Series Report No. 4). Stockholm: Stockholm Environment Institute.

Stack, C. 1974. *All Our Kin.* New York: Harper & Row.

Stephens, C. 1996. "Research on Urban Environmental Health." In *Urban Health Research in Developing Countries. Implications for Policy,* ed. S. Atkinson, J. Songsore, E. Werna. Wallingford: Cab International, pp. 115–134.

Stephens, C., Masamu, E.T., Kiama, M.G., Keto, A.J., Kinenekejo, M., Ichimori, K., Lines , J. 1995. "Knowledge of Mosquitoes in Relation to Public and Domestic Control Activities in the Cities of Dar es Salaam and Tonga." *Bulletin of the World Health Organization* 73(1): 97–104.

Stren, R.E. 1989a. "Urban Local Government in Africa." In *African Cities in Crisis. Managing Rapid Urban Growth,* ed. R.E. Stren, R.R. White. Boulder (San Francisco), London: Westview Press, pp. 20–36.

Stren, R.E. 1989b. "The Administration of Urban Services." In *African Cities in Crisis. Managing Rapid Urban Growth,* ed. R.E. Stren, R.R. White. Boulder (San Francisco), London: Westview Press, pp. 37 – 67.

Stren, R.E., White, R.R., eds. 1989. *African Cities in Crisis. Managing Rapid Urban Growth.* Boulder (San Francisco) and London: Westview Press.

Strittmatter, R. 1995. *Alltagswissen über Gesundheit und gesundheitliche Protektivfaktoren.* Frankfurt a.M.: Peter Lang.

Sutton, J.E.G. 1970. "Dar es Salaam. A Sketch of a Hundred Years." *Tanzania Notes and Records* 71: 1–19.

Svendsen, K. E. 1995. "Development Strategy and Crisis Management." In *Mwalimu. The Influence of Nyerere*, ed. C. Legum, G. Mmari. London: James Currey, pp. 108–124.

Svendsen, K. E., Teisen, M., eds. 1969. *Self-reliant Tanzania*. Dar es Salaam: Tanzania Publishing House.

Swantz, L. 1990. *The Medicine Man Among the Zaramo of Dar es Salaam*. Uppsala: Scandinavian Institute for African Studies in cooperation with the Dar es Salaam University Press.

Swantz, M.-L. 1986. *Ritual and Symbol in Transitional Zaramo Society with Special Reference to Women*. Uppsala: Scandinavian Institute of African Studies.

Swartz, M. 1991. *The Way the World Is. Cultural Processes and Social Relations Among the Mombasa Swahili*. Berkeley, Los Angeles and Oxford: University of California Press.

Swartz, M. 1997. "Illness and Morality in the Mombasa Swahili Community. A Metaphorical Model in an Islamic Culture." *Culture, Medicine, and Psychiatry* 21(1): 89–114.

Tabibzadeh, I., Rossi-Espagnet, A., Maxwell, R. 1989. *Spotlight on the Cities. Improving Urban Health in Developing Countries*. Geneva: World Health Organization.

Tanner, M., Vlassoff, C. 1998. "Treatment-seeking Behaviour for Malaria. A Typology Based on Endemicity and Gender." *Social Science and Medicine* 46.4/5: 523–532.

Tanzania Today, 1968. *A Portrait of the United Republic*. Nairobi: University Press of Africa.

Teisen, M. 1969. "Dar es Salaam." In *Self-reliant Tanzania*, ed. K. E. Svendsen, M. Teisen. Dar es Salaam: Tanzania Publishing House, pp.78–90.

Thurshen, M. 1984. *The Political Ecology of Disease in Tanzania*. New Brunswick: Rutgers University Press.

Tinker, I. ed. 1990 *Persistent Inequalities. Women and World Development*. New York, Oxford: Oxford University Press.

Trappe, P. 1966. "Afrikanischer Sozialismus." *Archiv für Rechts- und Sozialphilosophie* 52.3: 415–441. (nachgedruckt und aktualisiert In P. Trappe. 1984. *Entwicklungssoziologie*. Social Strategies, vol. 12. Basel: Soziologisches Seminar der Universität Basel, Karger Libri, pp. 261–279).

Trappe, P. 1984. *Entwicklungssoziologie* (Social Strategies, vol. 12.). Basel: Soziologisches Seminar der Universität Basel, Karger Libri.

Tripp, A. M. 1989. "Women and the Changing Household Economy in Urban Tanzania." *The Journal of Modern African Studies* 27(4): 601–623.

Tripp, A. M. 1992. "The Impact of Crisis and Economic Reform on Women in Urban Tanzania." In *Unequal Burden. Economic Crises, Persistent Poverty and Women's Work*, ed. L. Beneria, S. Feldman. Boulder: Westview Press, pp. 159–180.

Tripp, A.M. 1994. "Deindustrialization and the Growth of Women's Economic Associations and Networks in Urban Tanzania." In *Dignity and Daily Bread. New Forms of Economic Organising Among Poor Women in the Third World and the First*, ed. S. Rowbotham, S. Mitter. London, New York: Routledge, pp. 139–157.

Tripp, A.M. 1997. *Changing the Rules*. Berkeley: University of California Press.

Tungaraza, F. 1993. "Social Networks and Social Care in Tanzania." *Social Policy and Administration* 27(2): 141–150.

TzPPA (Tanzania Participatory Poverty Assessment) 2002/03. *Vulnerability and Resilience to Poverty in Tanzania. Causes, Consequences and Policy Implications. Main Report of Tanzania Participatory Poverty Assessment.* Dar es Salaam: The Economic and Social Research Foundation (E.S.R.F).

UN 2001. "The Chronicle Interview." *United Nations Chronicle (online edition)* 38.1. Available at: http://www.un.org/Pubs/chronicle/2001/issue1/0101p24.htm (2004, May 11).

UN 2004. *World Urbanization Prospects: The 2003 Revision.* Available at: http://www.unpopulation.org (2004, May 9).

UNCHS 1996. *An Urbanizing World. Global Report on Human Settlements 1996.* Oxford: Oxford University Press.

UN-Habitat 2002. *Dar es Salaam, Tanzania's trailblazer. UN-Habitat's Sustainable Cities Programme seeks improvements through participation.* Available at: http:www.unchs.org/mediacentre/wssd_pk5.asp (2003, July 10).

UN-Habitat 2003a. *The Challenge of Slums. Global Report on Human Settlements.* London: Earthscan.

United Republic of Tanzania 2003. *Poverty and Human Development Report.* Available at: http://www.tanzania.go.tz/pdf/PHDR_2003.pdf (2004, June 16).

United Republic of Tanzania 2004. Poverty *Reduction Strategy – Third Report.* Available at: http://www.tanzania.go.tz/pdf/THE%20THIRD%20PRSP%20Progress%20Report%202003.pdf (2004, July 16).

Vaughan, M. 1991. *Curing Their Ills. Colonial Power and African Illness.* Cambridge: Polity Press.

Vlassoff, C., Tanner, M. 1992. "The Relevance of Rapid Assessment to Health Research Interventions." *Health Policy and Planning* 7(1): 1–9.

Voipio, T., Hoebink, P. 1999. *European Aid for Poverty Reduction in Tanzania.* Helsinki: Institute of Development Studies.

Vorlaufer, K. 1973. *Dar es Salaam. Bevölkerung und Raum einer afrikanischen Grossstadt unter dem Einfluss von Urbanisierungs- und Mobilitätsprozessen* (Hamburger Beiträge zur Afrika-Kunde, 15). Hamburg: Deutsches Institut für Afrika-Forschung.

Watts, M. 2002. "Hour of Darkness. Vulnerability, Security and Globalization." *Geographica Helvetica* 57(1): 5–18.

Weiss, R. 2005. "Vulnerabilität und Resilienz aus transdisziplinärer Sicht." In: *Medizinethnologie im Spannungsfeld von Theorie und Praxis*, ed. P. van Eeuwijk, B. Obrist. Zürich: Seismo Verlag.

Werna, E., Harpham, T., Blue, I., Goldstein, G. 1998. *Healthy City Projects in Developing Countries. An International Approach to Local Problems*. London: Earthscan.

Whitehead, A. 1981. "I'm Hungry Mum: the Politics of Domestic Budgeting." In *Of Marriage and the Market*, ed. K. Young, C. Wolkowitz, R. McCullagh. London: CSE Books, pp. 88–111.

WHO 1967. *Constitution of the WHO*. Geneva: WHO.

WHO 1993. *The Urban Health Crisis. Strategies for Health for All in the Face of Rapid Urbanization*. Geneva: World Health Organization.

Whyte, S. R. 1989. "Anthropological Approaches to African Misfortune. From Religion to Medicine." In *Culture, Experience and Pluralism. Essays on African Ideas of Illness and Healing*, ed. A. Jacobson-Widding, D. Westerlund. Uppsala: Acta Universitatis Upsaliensis (Uppsala Studies in Cultural Anthropology, 13), pp. 289–301.

Whyte, S. R., ed. 1997. *Questioning Misfortune. The Pragmatics of Uncertainty in Eastern Uganda*. Cambridge: Cambridge University Press.

Wilk, R. R. 1991. *Household Ecology. Economic Change and Domestic Life Among the Kekchi Maya in Belize*. Tucson: University of Arizona Press.

Williams, R. 1990. *A Protestant Legacy. Attitudes to Death and Illness Among Older Aberdonians*. Claredon: Oxford.

Wohl, A. S. 1983. *Endangered Lives. Public Health in Victorian Britain*. London: Methuen.

World Health Report 2002. *Reducing Risks, Promoting Healthy Life*. Geneva: World Health Organization.

World Bank 2004. *Tanzania – Country Brief*. Available at: http://web.worldbank.org (2004, April 27).

Yhdego, M. 1991. "Urban Environmental Degradation in Tanzania." *Environment and Urbanization* 3(1): 147–152.

Young, A. 1982. "The Anthropologies of Illness and Sickness." *Annual Review of Anthropology* 11: 257–285.

Young, T. K. 1986. "Socialist Development and Primary Health Care. The Case of Tanzania." *Human Organization* 45.2: 128–134.

Zola, I. 1972. "Medicine as an Institution of Social Control." *Sociological Review* 20: 487–504.

Appendix 1
Geographic and ethnic origin
of married women (N = 93) and their husbands

Wife		Husband	
Region	*Ethnic Group*	*Region*	*Ethnic Group*
Tanga	Zigua	Tanga	Zigua
	Sambaa	Tanga	Sambaa
	Digo	Tanga	Digo
	Zigua	Tanga	Bondei
	Bondei	Pemba	Pemba
	Sambaa	Tanga	Sambaa
	Zigua	Tanga	Zigua
	Bondei	[Ruvuma]	Digo
	Digo	Tanga	Digo
	Zigua	Tanga	Zigua
	Arab	Pemba	Arab
	Digo	Pwani	Zaramo
	Zigua	Tanga	Zigua
	Sambaa	Tanga	Sambaa
Pwani	Zaramo	Pwani	Zaramo
	Zaramo	Pwani	Zaramo
	Zaramo	Morogoro	Luguru
	Ndengereko	Lindi	Bisa
	Zaramo	Tanga	Digo
	Zaramo	Tanga	Digo
	Ndengereko	Pwani	Ndengereko
	Zaramo	Tabora	Nyamwezi
	Kerewe	Morogoro	Luguru
	Ndengereko	Pwani	Ndengereko
	Zaramo	Pemba	Pemba
	Zaramo	Pwani	Zaramo
	Zaramo	Dar es Salaam	Zaramo
	Zaramo	Ruvuma	Yao
	Arab	Kigoma	Indian
	Rufiji	Morogoro	Sagara
	Zaramo	Tanga	Digo
	Zaramo	Tanga	Sambaa

(ctd.)

Wife		Husband	
Region	*Ethnic Group*	*Region*	*Ethnic Group*
Dar es Salaam	Arab	Dar es Salaam	Arab
	Arab	Mwanza	Arab
	Shihiri	Pemba	Pemba
	Zaramo	Dar es Salaam	Zaramo
	Zaramo	Dar es Salaam	Zaramo
	Indian	Mwanza	Indian
	Ngazija	Mbeya	Nyakusa
Lindi	Mwera	Pwani	Zaramo
	Ngindo	Lindi	Yao
	Ngindo	Pwani	Zaramo
	Nyasa	Mtwara	Manda
	Nyasa	Tanga	Bondei
Mtwara	Makua / Arab	Tabora	Nyamwesi / Arab
	Makonde	Rukwa	Fipa
Zanzibar	Arab	Zanzibar	Arab
Pemba	Pemba	Pemba	Pemba
	Pemba	Pemba	Pemba
	Pemba / Arab	Pemba	Pemba
	Pemba / Arab	Pemba	Pemba
	Pemba	Pemba	Pemba
Singida	Nyisanzu	Mwanza	Zinza
	Nyiramba	Pwani	Zaramo
Tabora	Nyamwezi	Pemba	Pemba
	Nyamwezi	Tanga	Digo
	Haya	Tabora	Haya
	Nyamwezi	Lindi	Mwera
Kigoma	Manyema	Singida	Nyiramba
	Ha	Pwani	Ndengereko
	Manyema	Mwanza	Kerewe
Kazera	Haya	Tanga	Digo
	Haya	Mwanza	Kerewe

(ctd.)

Wife		Husband	
Region	*Ethnic Group*	*Region*	*Ethnic Group*
Morogoro	Luguru	Kilimanjaro	Pare
	Pogoro	Tanga	Bondei
	Pogoro	Kilimanjaro	Chagga
	Vidunda	Pwani	Ndengereko
	Vidunda	Morogoro	Vidunda
	Luguru	Morogoro	Luguru
	Pogoro	Lindi	Makua
	Luguru	Morogoro	Pogoro
	Pogoro	Tanga	Zigua
	Kaguru	Morogoro	Kaguru
	Luguru	Morogoro	Luguru
	Sagara	Kilimanjaro	Chagga
Iringa	Manda	Iringa	Manda
	Hehe	Morogoro	Kutu
	Bena	Kilimanjaro	Chagga
Mbeya	Nyakusa	Ruvuma	Ngoni
	Nyakusa	Dar es Salaam	Zaramo
Ruvuma	Ngoni	Tanga	Digo
	Yao	Tanga	Digo
	Ngoni	Morogoro	Luguru
	Ngoni	Morogoro	Kutu
Rukwa	Fipa	Lindi	Ngindo
Kilimanjaro	Chagga	Kilimanjaro	Chagga
	Chagga	Kilimanjaro	Chagga
	Chagga	Morogoro	Mbunga
	Chagga	Morogoro	Pare
	Chaga	Mtwara	Makonde
	Chagga	Mtwara	Makonde
	Chagga	Mbeya	Sangu
	Pare	Morogoro	Mbunga
Kenya	–	Kilimanjaro	Chagga

Appendix 2
Social characteristics of wives and husbands in sub-sample (N = 20)

	Name	Ethnic Group	Grown up in/ Length of Stay	Religion	Education	Occupation
Wife	Tali	Nyisanzu	Lived in DSM all her life	Moslem	High School, Teachers' College	Primary School Teacher Sells ice cream
Husband		Zinza	Grown up in village, has lived in DSM since 1972	Moslem	Primary School	Clerk at the harbor
Wife	Agnes	Manda	Grown up in village, has lived in DSM since 1978	Christian	Primary School	Housewife
Husband		Manda	Grown up in village, has lived in DSM since 1968	Christian	Primary School	UNICEF Driver
Wife	Zawadi	Manyema	Grown up in Ujiji, has lived in DSM since 1980	Moslem	Primary School	Sells embroidery
Husband		Nyiramba	Lived in DSM all his life	Moslem	Primary School	Clerk at City Council
Female Headed Household	Zainab	Bondei	Grown up in town, has lived in DSM since 1969	Moslem	Primary School	Sells fish
Wife	Salima	Mwera	Lived in DSM all her life (born in Ilala, grown up in Temeke)	Moslem	Primary School	Keeps ducks, Employs tailors, Sells second-hand clothes
Husband		Zaramo	Lived in DSM all his life	Moslem	Primary School	Bus driver
Wife	Leticia	Pogoro	Grown up in village, has lived in DSM since 1980	Christian	Primary School	Sells food and fish
Husband		Bondei	Does not know –	Moslem	Does not know	Taylor
Wife	Johari	Hehe	Grown up in town, has lived in DSM since 1978/79	Moslem	Primary School	Housewife
Husband		Kutu	Lived in DSM all his life	Moslem	Primary School	Sells prawns from DSM in Nairobi

	Name	Ethnic Group	Grown up in/ Length of Stay	Religion	Education	Occupation
Wife	Farida	(Pemba)	Grown up in town, has lived in DSM since 1966	Moslem	Primary School	Housewife
Husband		(Pemba)	Grown up in town, has lived in DSM longer than his wife	Moslem	Primary School	Sells cars from Arab countries
Wife	Zubeda	Makua/ Arab	Grown up in town, has lived in DSM since 1984/85	Moslem	Primary School	Sells music cassettes from DSM in Zambia
Husband		Nyamwezi/ Arab	Grown up in village	Moslem	High School	Car mechanic
Wife	Telezea	Makonde	Grown up in village (Tanga), has lived in DSM since 1982	Christian	Primary School	Housewife
Husband		Fipa	Lived in DSM all his life	Christian	Primary School	Makes seat covers
Wife	Mariamu	(Pemba)	Grown up in village (Pemba), has lived in DSM since 1980/81	Moslem	High School	Housewife (stopped working)
		(Pemba)	Grown up in town (Pemba), has lived in DSM for very long time	Moslem	Moslem School	Sells French fries
Wife	Helena	Ngoni	Grown up in Mwanza town, has lived in DSM since 1978	Christian	Primary School	Sells peanuts
Husband		Luguru	Grown up in village, has lived in DSM since 1982	Christian	Primary School	Electrician
Wife	Ashura	Ndengereko	Lived in DSM all her life	Moslem	No School	Sells cooked food
Husband		Zaramo	Lived in DSM all his life	Moslem	Primary School	Retired clerk
Wife	Kalista	Luguru	Grown up in village, has been living in DSM since 1978	Christian	Primary School Teacher's College	Primary school teacher, has food garden, runs tuition classes
Husband		Luguru	Grown up in village, has been living in DSM since 1978	Christian	High School	Watchman

	Name	Ethnic Group	Grown up in/ Length of Stay	Religion	Education	Occupation
Wife	Salma	Zaramo	Has been living in DSM since 1974/75	Moslem	–	Sells chapati
Husband		Pemba	Grown up in Pemba, has been living in DSM since 1984/85	Moslem	Does not know	Taxi-driver
Female Headed Household	Rebeka	Nyakusa	Grown up in village, has been living in DSM since 1977	Christian	Primary School & Teachers Course	Secretary
Wife	Thecla	Bena	Grown up in Arusha, has been living in DSM since 1985/86	Christian	High School	Housewife
Husband		Chagga	Grown up in village, has been living in DSM since before 1984/85	Christian	Does not know	Business man
Wife	Clara	Saghala	Grown up and has lived in DSM all her life	Christian	High School	Keeps chicken
Husband		Chagga	Grown up in village, has been living in DSM since 1976	Christian	High School	Taxi driver, car mechanic
Wife	Mwajuma	Zaramo	Grown up and has been living in DSM for all of her life	Moslem	Primary School	Housewife (stopped working)
Husband		Digo	Grown up in village, has been living in DSM since 1984/85	Moslem	High School	Railway controller
Female Headed household	Beatrice	Pare	Grown up in village, has been living in DSM since 1987	Christian	High School	Secretary

Index

Adult Mortality and Morbidity Project 66–67, 104, 107, 114

Agency 19, 22, 41–44, 62, 262, 267, 300, 315; and structure 42, 44, 60, 144, 169, 173, 325; vs. coping 268; agents or actors 19, 22, 35, 41–44, 129, 145, 174, 225

Anthropology 19, 62, 65, 328; medical anthropology 21–22, 30, 61, 311; urban anthropology 21–22, 54; health anthropology 30–31, 61, 312

Antonovsky, Aaron 25, 62, 268, 324

Asset-Vulnerability-Framework 56–57, 60

Basic needs: in health explanations 136–137, 140; strategy 137; in health activities 145–146, 168, 169, 263, 283

Body: state or condition 129–133, 313; shape 130, 141, 143; image 131, 173

Bongoland 91, 328

Bourdieu, Pierre 19, 42–43, 62, 315

BP (blood pressure) 159

Burke, Timothy 34–35, 137, 313

Care 136, 138–140, 145, 302; as health activity 156–167, 263, 276

Chambers, Robert 54–55, 57, 261

Chant, Sylvia 47–49, 54, 59, 106–107, 217, 318

Child care 151, 199–205, 243–245, 265, 272–273, 278, 283, 288, 313, 318

Cleanliness (see also hygiene) in health definition 136; in health explanation 137–138, 140, 145, 169; in health activities 148–155, 265, 269, 282–283, 291, 313, 318; of the room 148, 196, 293, 298; of clothes 149–150, 196, 288, 293, 297; of the body 151; of the environment 152, 265, 289, 291, 293; of cooking utensils 153, 196, 293; control of pests 153–154, 291; 298, fresh air 154–155; household organization 194–198; fetching water 194–196

Commoditization 23, 56, 147, 172, 261, 306, 318

Contingencies 20, 23, 55, 224, 261, 308–309, 317

Dar es Salaam 11, 15–17, 21, 23, 66; Swahili settlement and colonial capital 72–73; capital of new socialist state 73–79; population growth 76–77; reforms 85–89; partial recovery 89–91; municipalities 89, 240, 329; threats of urban development 261

Dar es Salaam Urban Health Project 11, 66, 89

Decision-making 21, 50–51, 65, 176, 258, 271, 273, 277, 279, 290, 292, 294, 295, 329

Diarrhea 161–163, 280, 299

Douglas, Mary 28–29, 42, 51, 176

Dysentery 163

Environmental hazards 18, 23, 56, 172, 261, 306, 317–318; decline in services 81; in Ilala Ilala 122, 172

Faith (see also trust) 160, 164, 174, 224

Faltermaier, Toni 39–40, 64, 127, 169, 312–313, 315

Food: provision 141, 145–147, 170, 272, 313, 318; paying for food 186–188, 275–276; buying food 189–190, 273, 275–276, 290, 292; cooking food 190–192, 265, 278, 282, 288, 293, 298; food gifts 186, 189, 212, 226, 249; food for heard times 283

Foucault, Michel 19, 35, 36, 43–44, 172, 315

Garbage (or waste): in health explanations 138; and children 164, 203

Garbage (or waste) removal 17–18, 56, 68; in Dar es Salaam 81, 99, 251, 257, 317; privatization 87–90, 99; as health activity 155–156, 222, 235–240, 242, 250, 265, 319–321; improvements 329

Generating income: as health activity 178–185, 313; women not involved 290–291, 297; women involved 269, 271–289, 292, 295–296; as contested value 301; as health activity 313; as response option 263–264, 318; as women's empowerment 329

Gender: in division of labor 20, 48–50; differential risks 20; relations 21; division of responsibilities 23, 35, 48–50, 68, 175, 177–178, 192, 225, 247; in concepts of health 38; models vs. relations 49, 68, 176; negotiation 50–51, 176, inequality 51, 218–219, 321; in health practice 64; changes in relations 92–93, 320; gender models and relations in Ilala Ilala 117–122, 213, 218, 263, 266, 300, 302, 320, 323; productive and reproductive work 175, 177, 179–185, 192, 216, 263, 265–266, 275, 279, 281, 296, 298, 321; negotiating responsibilities 177, 188, 211, 218, 321, 329; help vs.

responsibility 187, 215, 218, 220, 230

Giddens, Anthony 19, 41, 43, 62, 128, 144, 315, 326

González de la Rocha, Mercedes 47, 52, 54, 175, 221, 318

Governance: corruption 94; culture of non-compliance 94

Hannerz, Ulf 19, 36

Hansen, Karen Tranberg 47, 53; 104, 221, 318

Harpham, Trudy 15–18, 20–21, 61, 147, 170, 317

Healers 159–160, 167, 183

Health: epidemiological transition 16–17; as a value 25; Western definitions 25, 36–40; health promotion 25; public health 26, 34, 56, 61, 174, 312, 317; health behavior 28–31, 40, 45; health as social experience 42–43, 170, 268; good health 30, 64; 173; Swahili concepts of good health *(afya nzuri, uzima)* 133, 169, 170, 313, 317, 325; notions of balance 31–33, 37; health vs. illness conceptions 37, 311–312; positive and negative dimensions 38, 45, 134, 311, 312; health concepts 39–40; health theories 39–40; health action 39–40; health production 45; health maintenance 45; as human capital 57–58; Swahili term for health *(afya)* 76, 127, 171; health in the home *(afya nyumbani)* 127, 140, 170, 175, 216, 220, 314; health development 138, 171–173, 263, 312–313, 315; public health knowledge 263, 313, 315, 323, 326

Health care: health care services 90; in Ilala Ilala 103; as health activity 158–160, 265, 266, 313, 318; gen-

356

dered responsibilities 205–210, 302; decision making dynamics 207–210; beyond the household 245–248;

Health education: Mass mobilization campaign *Mtu ni Afya* 75, 171, 314; for children 164–166

Health practice 21–23, 41, 49, 59, 88, 175, 221, 257, 270, 318, 326, 328; health definitions 42, 129–135; 169, 312–313, 326; health explanations 42, 135–145, 169, 312–313, 326; health activities 42, 45, 68, 145–169, 175, 262, 280, 312–313, 318, 326; framework 63; health conceptions 63, 127; social organization 64, 184, 216; links with vulnerability 61, 65, 140, 174, 328; health notions 68; preventive measures 166–167; health protection 167; health and urban life 169–170

Herzlich, Claudine 26, 36–38, 40, 61, 127, 312, 313, 315

HIV/Aids 55, 130, 283, 296, 298

Hoodfar, Homa 47–48, 50, 52–53, 175, 188, 218, 221, 318, 320

Household: diverse household conditions 18; headship 21, 68; as socio-spatial construct 21; internal dynamics 23; as arena 44, 318; household health production 45, 140, 170, 172, 216; definitions 45–47; feminist critique 46–53; urban structures 47–48, 68, 179; female headship 47, 59, 106–107, 267, 272, 284, 287, 295; decision making 50; and social networks 51; effects of reforms 88; structures in Ilala Ilala 104–07, 319; headship in Ilala Ilala 117–122, 184–185, 218, 271, 273, 277, 281, 290, 292, 297, 320; as safety net 220

Humoral traditions: in Europe, Asia, Latin America and Africa 31; in Mombasa 32, 170, 314; in Dar es Salaam 171, 314

Hygiene (see also cleanliness) 26, 45: hygiene behavior 28–29, 31; in Zimbabwe 34; training and domesticity 34–35, 137, 170–171, 314; in health explanations 140, 145; teaching children 164–166; in health activities 151, 168, 263, 266, 272, 326–327

Ilala: name 95–98; history 98–99; population 99; ethnicity 107–113; collective identities 113–117

Janzen, John M. 32, 34

Krüger, Fred 55, 58–59, 79, 261, 308

Livelihood 54: concept 55; and vulnerability 58; in Dar es Salaam 95; living conditions *(hali ya maisha)* 136, 297, 313

Lock, Margaret 36, 134, 173–174, 305, 327

Lomnitz, Larissa 51–52, 54, 93, 222, 258

Lugalla, Joe 73, 77–85, 91–95, 98, 116, 221–222

Malaria 55, 278; malaria prevention 156–158, 168; mosquito-malaria link 157–158; treatment 210, 274, 282–283, 291, 293

Massé, Raymond 31, 61, 311

Medicalization 35, 173, 300, 316, 326

Middleton, John 111, 124

Mind: state of the mind 129, 133–134, 313

Mkapa, Benjamin 89

Morality: moral subjects 22, 43, 172; moral judgments 44, 166; moral convictions 164, 167; in gender relations 213; help as moral obligation 307, 322–323

Moser, Caroline 46–47, 50, 52, 56–57, 60, 93, 147, 172, 185, 217, 219, 221, 261, 306–307, 317, 320

Mwinyi, Ali Hassan 85

Negotiations: beyond the household 277

Nyerere, Julius 73–74, 85, 124, 137, 171, 314

Omari, C. K. 75, 92, 93, 95, 105–107, 112

Practice 19, 41–44, 60, 62, 129, 161, 169, 263, 315

Poverty: urbanization of poverty 16, 85; health and poverty 19, 23; critique of the concept 54–55; poverty categories in Ilala 116–117

Reciprocity: generalized vs. balanced 255–256, 259, 286–287, 322

Resilience 22–23, 59, 65, 262, 306, 308, 324; vs. coping 268, 324–328, 329

Response options to health risks 22–23, 59–60, 261–268, 306, 318, 323–326

Risk: synergy 16, 18; urban environment 20, 22–23, 26, 261–262, 316, 318, 324; perception 28–29; definition 62

Salutogenic idea 25, 62, 268, 324

Sahlins. Marshall 286, 322

Sanitation 17, 26, 34–35, 45, 56, 68, 122–123, 317, 319–321: sanitary idea 27; sanitation related diseases 28; sewerage 18, 27, 81, 90, 99, 315; privatization 87–90; cesspit emptying 239, 240–243, 250, 265, 289; improvements 329

Slum 84

Slum Clearance Program 78; in Ilala 98–99, 194, 227, 240

Social capital 57

Social fragmentation 23, 56, 172, 261, 306, 318

Social networks 21, 23: definition 51; social solidarity 52, 230, 239, 303; access to resources 53, 265, 323; ideology of assistance 93, 222, 253, 258; safety nets 221, 259; ROSCAs 256, 285, 300–301; single- vs. multi-stranded networks 303; romantization 323; act of balance 328

Social organization of health practice: in income generation 178–185, 223–225; in food provision 185–193, 225–226; in cleanliness 194–198, 227; in child care 199–205, 243–245; in health care 205–211, 245–248

Songsore, Jacob 17–18

Support 176: receiving support 211–215, 248–251, 273, 275, 277, 278, 291, 295, 297, 322; giving support 251–253, 265–267, 272, 274, 279, 282, 297; reciprocity and support 220, 253–256, 259, 286–287, 308; help vs. responsibility 186–187, 194, 215, 218, 220, 230, 245, 250, 259–260, 265, 286–287, 289, 307, 320, 322; contributions in money (*kuchangia*) 232, 250, 319; contributions in labour (*zamu*) 234–235, 250, 319; gifts 254, 294, 304; mobilizing support 263, 265, 267, 270, 299, 321, 323; as a complex value 302; moral and practical support 303

Survival strategies 22, 52, 54, 175; culture of non-compliance 94

Swahili: coast 30, 105; in Mombasa 32, 111; towns 72; culture 72–73, 171, 245, 314; house 99–103, 114, 214, 232, 236, 240, 242, 257–258, 269, 271, 273, 277, 280, 281, 284, 287, 290, 292, 295, 297, 307; identity and ethnicity 108–113, 124; in

Zanzibar and Lamu 113; gender model 178; values 192; 218–219; house community 235–236, 265, 319

Swartz, Marc J. 30, 32, 111, 127, 314

Swantz, Lloyd 30, 127

Swantz, Marja-Liisa 30, 127

Tanner, Marcel 16, 20,

Tanzania Participatory Poverty Assessment 55, 59–60, 91, 93–94, 116, 123, 173, 261, 316

Task-centered interactions 64, 175–176, 222, 225, 318

Tripp, Aili Mari 85–86, 91–93, 115, 123, 175, 221, 224, 319, 321

Trust (see also faith): in medical knowledge 43–44; deriving from social ties 57, 271; in water safety 160, 162, 221; in prayers 167, 174; in food vendors 280; in boyfriend 288; in God 299; between researcher and study participants 305; in fellow-tenants 307; sources of information 316, 329

Tungaraza, Felician 91, 93

Typhoid 162–163

Tuberculosis (TB) 269

Urban health crisis 15–16, 22, 27, 49, 56, 65: in Dar es Salaam 79–85, 88; in Ilala Ilala 102, 123, 175, 261, 269

Vulnerability 22–23, 54, 261: concept 55–56, 62, 317–318; urban vulnerability 56–57, 172, 306, 317; asset-vulnerability framework 56–57; and livelihood 58–59; to poverty 59–60; to health risks 61, 174; health and vulnerability 65; as personal and social experience 144; dynamic dimensions 262, 308, 327; degrees 266, 323; least vulnerable 266, 269–279, 305; middle group 266–267, 280–289, 305; most vulnerable 267, 290–299, 305

Waste-water-complex 68

Water: inadequate water supply 17–18, 57, 81, 84, 94–95, 174, 317, 320; move towards privatization 87–91; water supply in Ilala Ilala 98–99, 122, 177, 227–233, 257, 284, 291, 315, 320, 321; as prerequisite for health 136–140, 148, 169, 291, 325; for laundry 149–50, 293; for personal hygiene 151, 199, 205; for clean home environment 152–153, 234; boiling water 139, 160–163, 173, 212, 274, 280, 288–289, 313, 316, 327; water-borne illness 28, 162, 320; fetching water 168, 194–196, 214, 222, 227–233, 249–250, 274, 280, 284, 298, 306–307, 319–321; dirty water 203–204, 241–243, 289, 291; water bills 250, 281; clean or safe water 258, 278, 313, 320, 327; improvements in water provision 258, 329

Well-being 33, 39, 56, 60–61, 133–134, 317, 323

Worms 163, 167

Whyte, Susan Reynolds 33, 34